VERTEBRAL AUGMENTATION TECHNIQUES

Other books in this series

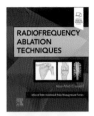

Alaa Abd-Elsayed, Radiofrequency Ablation Techniques, 1e
ISBN: 9780323870634

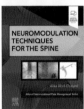

Alaa Abd-Elsayed, Neuromodulation Techniques for the Spine, 1e
ISBN: 9780323875844

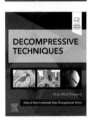

Alaa Abd-Elsayed, Decompressive Techniques, 1e
ISBN : 9780323877510

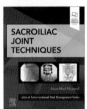

Alaa Abd-Elsayed, Sacroiliac Joint Techniques, 1e
ISBN: 9780323877541

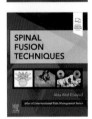

Alaa Abd-Elsayed, Spinal Fusion Techniques, 1e
ISBN: 9780323882231

VERTEBRAL AUGMENTATION TECHNIQUES

Atlas of Interventional Pain Management Series

Alaa Abd-Elsayed, MD, MPH, CPE, FASA

Medical Director, UW Health Pain Services
Medical Director, UW Pain Clinic
Division Chief, Chronic Pain Management
Department of Anesthesiology
University of Wisconsin
Madison, Wisconsin
United States

ELSEVIER

Elsevier
1600 John F. Kennedy Blvd.
Ste 1800
Philadelphia, PA 19103-2899

VERTEBRAL AUGMENTATION TECHNIQUES
ATLAS OF INTERVENTIONAL PAIN MANAGEMENT SERIES   ISBN: 978-0-323-88226-2

Notice

Practitioners and researchers must always rely on their own experience and knowledge in evaluating
and using any information, methods, compounds, or experiments described herein. Because of rapid
advances in the medical sciences, in particular, independent verification of diagnoses and drug dosages
should be made. To the fullest extent of the law, no responsibility is assumed by Elsevier, authors, editors,
or contributors for any injury and/or damage to persons or property as a matter of products liability,
negligence or otherwise, or from any use or operation of any methods, products, instructions, or ideas
contained in the material herein.

Senior Content Development Manager: Somodatta Roy Choudhury
Executive Content Strategist: Michael Houston
Senior Content Development Specialist: Malvika Shah
Publishing Services Manager: Shereen Jameel
Project Manager: Vishnu T. Jiji
Senior Designer: Patrick C. Ferguson

Printed in India

Last digit is the print number: 9 8 7 6 5 4 3 2 1

Working together
to grow libraries in
developing countries

www.elsevier.com • www.bookaid.org

To my parents, wife, and my two beautiful kids, Maro and George

Contributors

Alaa Abd-Elsayed, MD, MPH, CPE, FASA
Medical Director, UW Health Pain Services
Medical Director, UW Pain Clinic
Division Chief, Chronic Pain Management
Department of Anesthesiology
University of Wisconsin
Madison, Wisconsin
United States

Mohammad H. Bawany, MD
Department of Emergency Medicine
University of Wisconsin School of Medicine and
    Public Health
Madison, Wisconsin
United States

Clayton Busch, MD
Department of Anesthesiology
The Ohio State University, Wexner Medical Center
Columbus, Ohio
United States

Ahish Chitneni, DO
Department of Rehabilitation and Regenerative
    Medicine
New York-Presbyterian Hospital -Columbia and
    Cornell
New York, New York
United States

Pooja Chopra, MD
Pain Management Physician
Bux Pain Management
Danville, Kentucky
United States

Kenneth J. Fiala, BS
University of Wisconsin School of Medicine and
    Public Health
Madison, Wisconsin
United States

Gabrielle Frisenda, MD
Department of Anesthesia and Critical Care
University of Chicago
Chicago, Illinois
United States

Manuchehr Habibi, MD
Department of Anesthesiology
University of Wisconsin School of Medicine and
    Public Health
Madison, Wisconsin
United States

Nasir Hussain, MD, MSc
Department of Anesthesiology
The Ohio State University, Wexner Medical Center
Columbus, Ohio
United States

Navdeep S. Jassal, MD
Assistant Clinical Professor
Department of Neurology/Pain
University of South Florida
Tampa, Florida
United States

Ahmed Malik
University of Chicago
Chicago, Illinois
United States

Tariq Malik, MD
Associate Professor
Anesthesia and Critical Care
University of Chicago
Chicago, Illinois
United States

Genevieve Marshall, DO
Department of Physical Medicine and Rehabilitation
Zucker School of Medicine at Hofstra/Northwell
  Health
Long Island, New York
United States

Joshua M. Martens, BS
University of Wisconsin School of Medicine and
  Public Health
Madison, Wisconsin
United States

David J. Mazur-Hart, MD
Department of Neurological Surgery
Oregon Health & Science University
Portland, Oregon
United States

Kailash Pendem, MD
Department of Physical Medicine and Rehabilitation
University of Florida
Gainesville, Florida
United States

Keth Pride, MD
Assistant Professor
Department of Anesthesiology
University of Wisconsin School of Medicine and
  Public Health
Madison, Wisconsin
United States

Ahmed M. Raslan, MD
Vice Chair for Clinical Affairs
Department of Neurological Surgery
Oregon Health & Science University
Portland, Oregon
United States

Lucas Vannoy, DO
Department of Anesthesiology
University of Wisconsin School of Medicine and
  Public Health
Madison, Wisconsin
United States

Ognjen Visnjevac, MD
Chief, Spine Pain Program, Bloor Pain Specialists
Anesthesiologist & Pain Management Physician,
  Cleveland Clinic Canada and Bloor Pain Specialists;
Assistant Clinical Professor (Adjunct)
Department of Anesthesiology
Faculty of Health Sciences
McMaster University
Hamilton, Ontario
Canada

Nasser K. Yaghi, MD
Department of Neurological Surgery
Oregon Health & Science University
Portland, Oregon
United States

Preface

Vertebral augmentation is an advanced procedure performed by pain physicians, interventional radiologists, and spine surgeons. Over time, revolutionary changes in equipment, technique, and equipment have dramatically altered the performance of these procedures.

Vertebral augmentation is a profoundly critical procedure that requires thoughtful patient selection and a thorough understanding of procedural indications, contraindications, and optimal maximization of improvements in procedural outcomes.

This book provides a definitive guide for practitioners performing vertebral augmentation, incorporating detailed figures and perspectives from leaders in the field to maximize the conveyance of currently practiced techniques.

I would like to thank the authors and publisher for their support and dedication in bringing this guide to practitioners.

Alaa Abd-Elsayed, MD, MPH, CPE, FASA

Contents

Chapter 1

Vertebral Anatomy

Mohammad H. Bawany, Ognjen Visnjevac, and Alaa Abd-Elsayed

A detailed understanding of spinal anatomy is requisite to performing spinal procedures. The spine consists of bones, ligaments, discs, blood vessels, and nerves.

Bony Structures and Ligaments of the Spine

The bony components of the spine, or vertebrae, begin at the transition from the skull to the cervical spine, also known as the *craniocervical junction*. In total, 33 bones make up the entire vertebral column. Of these bones, 24 are individually separate though linked to each other through joints and ligaments to provide both support and flexibility. The lower nine bones are fused in adults and make up the sacrum and coccyx (Fig. 1.1).[1] This chapter will focus on the upper 24 vertebrae.

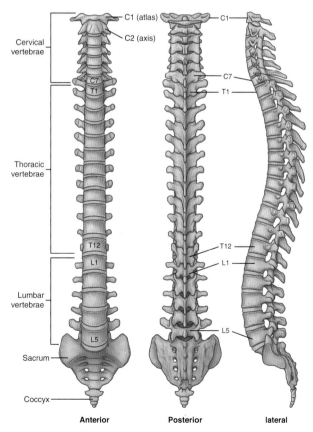

Cervical vertebrae
C1 (atlas)
C2 (axis)
C7
T1

Thoracic vertebrae
C1
C7
T1

T12
L1

Lumbar vertebrae
T12
L1
L5

Sacrum
L5

Coccyx

Anterior   Posterior   lateral

Fig. 1.1 Anterior, posterior, and lateral views of bony structures of the spine. (From Cleveland Clinic Center for Medical Art & Photography © 2011–2015. All rights reserved. With permission.)

The upper 24 vertebrae can be divided into 7 cervical, 12 thoracic, and 5 lumbar. Accurate and consistent numbering of vertebrae is critical in guiding interventions. Therefore, it is important to note anatomical variants that may be encountered, including L5 sacralization, which is incorporation of the L5 vertebral body into the sacrum (Fig. 1.2).[2]

The vertebrae are arranged such that, when in the upright position, they make naturally occurring curves. These curves assist in the spine's ability to

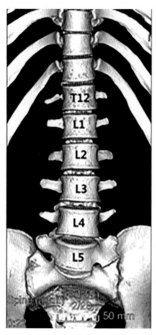

Fig. 1.2 Sacralization. L5 fuses fully or partially into the sacrum, on one or both sides. Sacralization is a congenital anomaly. (From Doo AR, Lee J, Yeo GE, et al. The prevalence and clinical significance of transitional vertebrae: a radiologic investigation using whole spine spiral three-dimensional computed tomographic images. *Anesth Pain Med.* 2020;15(1):103-110, Fig. 2.)

distribute vertical compressive forces. When viewed from the side, the cervical and lumbar spines appear concave, known as *lordosis*, whereas the thoracic spine appears convex, known as *kyphosis* (Fig. 1.3).[3]

While there are structural variations, most of the vertebrae are composed of an anterior part and a posterior part. The anterior part of a vertebra contains the vertebral body. Externally, it is made of a hard shell of compact bone; internally, it consists of

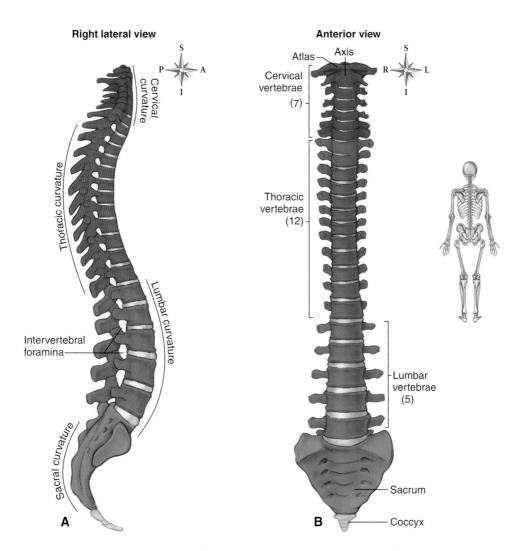

Fig. 1.3 Natural curvature of the spine. (From Patton K, Thibodeau G, Douglas M. *Essentials of Anatomy and Physiology.* Elsevier; 2012: 161, Fig. 9.10.)

marrow-containing trabecular bone, which is innervated by the sinuvertebral and basivertebral nerves (Fig. 1.4).[4]

Each vertebral body is separated by intervertebral discs that sit between adjacent vertebrae. These discs aid in load bearing and are discussed later. The posterior part of a vertebra contains the vertebral arch, which includes the pedicle, lamina, spinous process, transverse process, and superior and inferior articular processes, which form the facet or zygapophyseal joints (Fig. 1.5).[5]

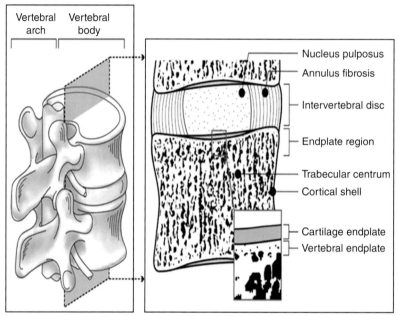

Fig. 1.4 Vertebral structure. (Left) A vertebra is split into the vertebral arch posteriorly and vertebral body anteriorly. (Right) The body is made up of trabecular bone surrounded by a cortical shell. Superiorly and inferiorly is the end-plate region, atop which sits the intervertebral disc. (Modified from Auger JD, Frings N, Wu Y, et al. Trabecular architecture and mechanical heterogeneity effects on vertebral body strength. *Curr Osteoporos Rep.* 2020;18:716-726, Fig. 1.)

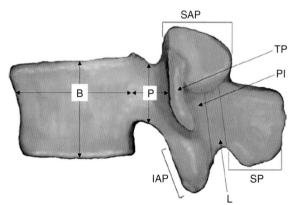

Fig. 1.5 Lumbar vertebra, superior view (*left*) and lateral view (*right*). B, Vertebral body; C, spinal canal; IAP, inferior articulating process; L, lamina; P, pedicle; PI, pars interarticularis; SAP, superior articulating process; SP, spinous process; TP, transverse process. (Modified from Manjila SV, Mroz, TE, Steinmetz MP. *Lumbar Interbody Fusions,* 1st ed. Elsevier; 2018. chap 3, 19-21, Figs. 3.1 and 3.2.)

The pedicles connect the vertebral body to the transverse processes as well as the laminae, together creating the arch, which helps encase the spinal cord. Nerve roots exit inferior to each pedicle; thus, the pedicle is a key anatomical landmark to identify during needle placement for interventional procedures.[6] With fluoroscopic imaging, pedicles appear as rounded areas of increased bone density (Fig. 1.6).[7]

The laminae connect the transverse processes to the spinous process and form the roof of the spinal canal through which the spinal cord travels. The spinous process is the point for muscle and ligament attachment, notably, those muscles used for extension of the vertebral column.[3] The articular processes also project from the laminae and allow a vertebra to articulate with the vertebrae above and below it to form the zygapophyseal, or facet, joints (Fig. 1.7).[8]

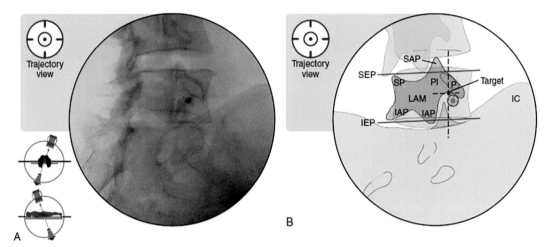

Fig. 1.6 The "Scotty dog" in lumbar oblique projections that assists in identifying fluoroscopic landmarks. (A) Fluoroscopic image with needle in position for a supra-neural transforaminal epidural steroid injection. (B) How the anatomical landmarks create the "Scotty dog" outline and eye. IAP, Inferior articular process—front and back legs; IEP, inferior endplate; LAM, lamina—body; P, pedicle—eye; PI, pars interarticularis—neck; SAP, superior articular process—ear; SEP, superior endplate; SP, spinous process—tail. (From Furman MB. *Atlas of Image-Guided Spinal Procedures.* 2nd ed. Elsevier; 2018:chap 3, 27-65, Fig. 3.20.)

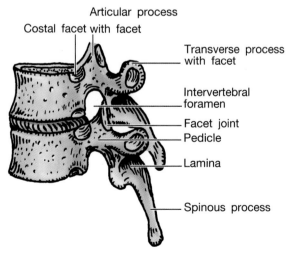

Fig. 1.7 Facet joints in lateral view. (From Mahadevan V. Anatomy of the vertebral column. *Surgery (Oxford).* 2018;36(7):327-332, Fig. 4.)

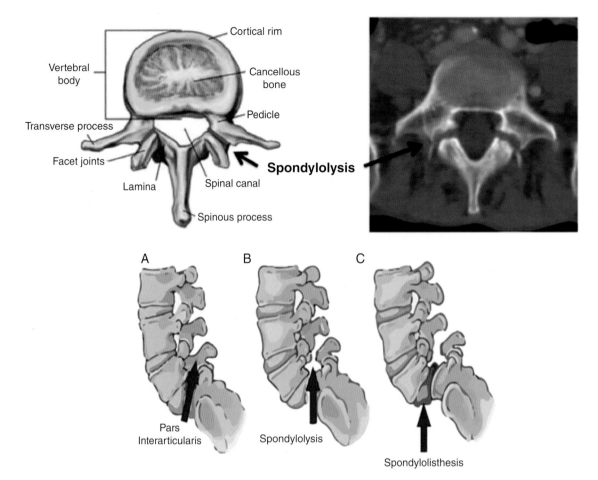

Fig. 1.8 Top (*left and right*) showing a defect in the pars interarticularis (PI), termed *spondylolysis*. Bottom showing sagittal views of the spine with the intact PI (A), pars defect (B), or spondylolysis, and anterior displacement of the L5 vertebral body (C), or spondylolisthesis. (Modified from Chakravarthy V, Patel A, Kemp W, Steinmetz M. Surgical treatment of lumbar spondylolisthesis in the elderly. *Neurosur Clin N Am.* 2019;30(3):341-352.)

The thicker portion of the lamina that acts as the junction connecting the spinous processes to the superior and inferior articular processes on a single vertebra is known as the *pars interarticularis*. It is prone to "pars defects," or fractures known as *spondylolysis*, which can lead to the displacement of a vertebral body, known as *spondylolisthesis* (Fig. 1.8). Spondylolisthesis can result in nerve root compression.[9]

Cervical Spine

The superior-most vertebra, C1, is termed the *atlas*. The second, C2, is termed the *axis* (Fig. 1.9).[10] Together, they account for most of the rotational ability of the cervical spine. C1 attaches the skull to the spine. It is unlike the other vertebrae in that it lacks a vertebral body and a spinous process. It is shaped like a ring: two lateral masses are connected by an anterior and posterior arch. The anterior arch comes to a midpoint that contains the dorsal facet, which allows for a connection with the dens on the vertebral body of C2, allowing C1 to pivot the skull.[11,12] The posterior arch of C1 contains the posterior tubercle at its midpoint, which serves as the origin for the rectus capitis posterior minor muscle, which assists head and neck extension.[3,10]

In the posterior portion of each posterior arch is a groove in which the vertebral artery and first cervical

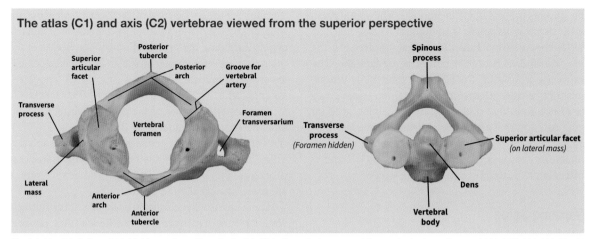

The atlas (C1) and axis (C2) vertebrae viewed from the superior perspective

Fig. 1.9 The C1 (*left*) and C2 (*right*) vertebrae. (From Bazira PJ. Clinically applied anatomy of the vertebral column. *Surgery.* 2021;39(6):315-323, Fig. 4.)

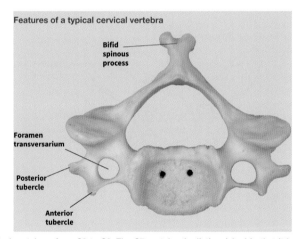

Features of a typical cervical vertebra

Fig. 1.10 Features of typical cervical vertebrae from C3 to C6. The C7 vertebra is distinguished in that it has a monofid spinous process and no foramen transversarium. (From Bazira PJ. Clinically applied anatomy of the vertebral column. *Surgery.* 2021;39(6):315-323, Fig. 3.)

spinal nerve are found. Injecting in this region can be technically challenging. The posterior cavity of the atlas formed by the anterior and posterior arches contains the spinal cord. The lateral masses of C1 contain the superior articular processes/facets that connect it to the occiput, or skull base, and inferior articular processes that connect it to C2.

The C2 vertebra, or the axis, is composed of a body that contains a vertical pillar of bone, the dens, which articulates with C1 above. The inferior facets are located at the junction of the pedicles and laminae.[10] The spinous process of C2 is bifid and provides a

prominent bony landmark for palpation. It is also the attachment for several suboccipital muscles and the ligamentum nuchae (nuchal ligament), which extends from the external occipital protuberance to the C7 spinous process.

The lower cervical vertebrae (C3–C7) adopt the more usual vertebral structure detailed previously, but they are distinguished (except for C7) by the presence of a perforation in each transverse process, termed the *foramen transversarium*, that transmits the vertebral artery and sympathetic plexuses (Fig. 1.10).[10] Further, the spinous processes of C3 to C6 are bifid, whereas the spinous process of C7 is monofid. The spinal canal of the cervical vertebrae is triangular; its anterior border is the vertebral body, its lateral borders are the pedicles, and its posterior border is the laminae. The transverse process in the cervical vertebrae is unique not only because it contains the foramen transversarium but also in that it gives off two tubercles, anterior and posterior, that attach the scalene muscles used for lateral neck flexion. The anterior tubercle of C6 is notable in that it is termed the *carotid tubercle* and is immediately posterior to the carotid artery.[3]

Thoracic Spine

The thoracic region is the least mobile area of the spine, partly due to stability provided by the rib cage and sternum. A primary function of the thoracic spine, in connection with the ribs and sternum, is protection of thoracic organs, including the heart and lungs. The bodies of the thoracic spine vertebrae are unique in that their upper and lower lateral borders house areas, known as *demi-facets*, for articulation with the heads of the ribs (Fig. 1.11).[13]

The posterior arches of the thoracic vertebrae contain the same components as those seen in Fig. 1.5: the vertebral foramen, pedicles, superior and inferior articular processes, spinous processes, and transverse processes. The spinous processes of thoracic vertebrae are more acutely slanted caudad.

There are usually 12 ribs on each side of the thoracic vertebra. Ribs 1 to 7 are true ribs in that they connect to the costal cartilage of the sternum anteriorly; ribs 8 to 12 are false ribs in that their costal cartilages are

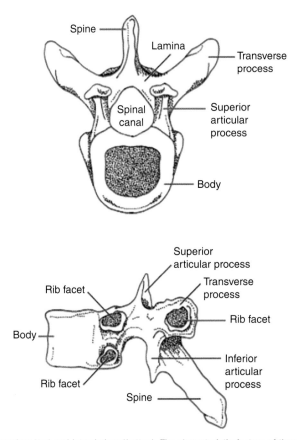

Fig. 1.11 Thoracic vertebra superior view (*top*) and lateral view (*bottom*). The characteristic feature of thoracic vertebrae is the presence of rib facets/demi-facets, joints that articulate with ribs. (GD Cramer, SA Darby Basic and clinical anatomy of the spine, spinal cord, and ANS (2nd ed.), Elsevier Mosby, St Louis (2005))

connected to the rib above. Ribs 11 and 12 are also floating ribs, which do not project anteriorly.

Lumbar Spine

Five vertebrae compose the lumbar portion of the spine. The vertebral bodies are large, and the posterior arch, formed by the pedicles, laminae, and articular processes, encloses the vertebral foramen. These vertebrae are unique in their lack of costal facets and foramen transversaria (Fig. 1.12). The

spinous processes are near horizontal, making for large interlaminar spaces that are easily visualized using a fluoroscopic approach during interventions (Fig. 1.13).[8,14]

Ligaments of the Spine

Ligaments of the spine, from most superficial to deep starting dorsally, are the supraspinous ligament, the interspinous ligament, the ligamentum flavum, the posterior longitudinal ligament, and the anterior longitudinal

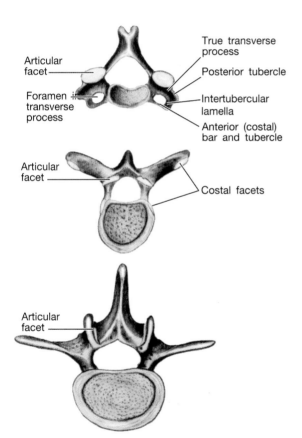

Fig. 1.12 Superior views of typical cervical (*top*), thoracic (*middle*), and lumbar (*bottom*) vertebrae. A common architectural design with unique variations can be appreciated. (From Mahadevan V. Anatomy of the vertebral column. *Surgery (Oxford)*. 2018;36(7):327-332, Fig. 2.)

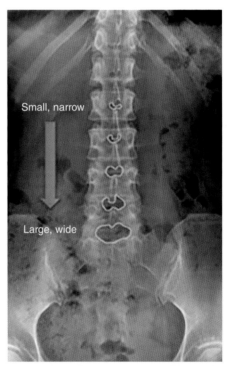

Fig. 1.13 Interlaminar window size and shape (*outlined in yellow*) of the lumbar vertebrae. Fluoroscopic views make it apparent that there is a noticeable size difference between the visibility of the thoracic and lumbar interlaminar windows. (From Shin KH. Percutaneous full-endoscopic interlaminar lumbar spine surgery. In: Kim J-S, Lee JH, Ahn Y, eds. *Endoscopic Procedures on the Spine*. Springer Singapore; 2020:chap 15, 185-209, Fig. 15.1.)

ligament (Fig. 1.14).[8] The supraspinous ligament is a fibrous band that joins the tips of the spinous processes and ends between L4 and L5. The interspinous ligaments connect adjacent spinous processes from roots to apices. The ligamentum flavum begins in C1 to C2 superiorly and extends to L5 to S1 inferiorly.[15] It connects adjacent laminae and forms the dorsal boundary of the epidural space. With age, the ligamentum flavum loses elasticity and thickens, potentially causing spinal canal stenosis.[16,17]

The posterior and anterior longitudinal ligaments are composed of layers; the deep layer connects adjacent vertebrae, whereas the superficial layers can extend fibers over three vertebrae. The posterior longitudinal ligament begins at C2 and extends inferiorly to the sacrum. It is fused to the posterior annulus fibrosis of the intervertebral discs, making up the anterior border of the spinal canal. A major function of this ligament is to prevent posterior disc herniation into the spinal canal. The anterior longitudinal ligament is

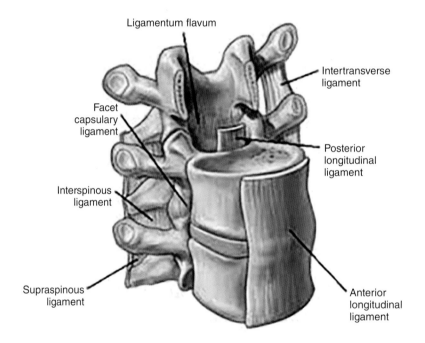

Fig. 1.14 Vertebral column showing vertebral ligaments. (*Left*) Bisected view showing the supraspinous ligament, interspinous ligament, and ligamentum flavum. (*Right*) Anterior view showing the supraspinous ligament, interspinous ligament, ligamentum flavum, posterior longitudinal ligament, and anterior longitudinal ligament. (Modified from Mahadevan V. Anatomy of the vertebral column. *Surgery (Oxford)*. 2018;36(7):327-332, Fig. 5.)

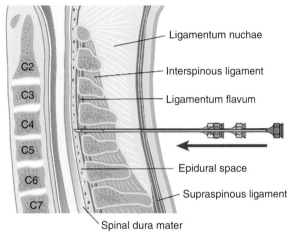

Fig. 1.15 Ligamentous anatomy of the cervical spine. With a needle inserted starting dorsally to access the epidural space, one would first encounter the supraspinous ligament, then the interspinous ligament, and the ligamentum flavum. (From Waldman S. *Atlas of Interventional Pain Management.* 4th ed. Elsevier; 2015:chap 45, 206, Fig. 45.5.)

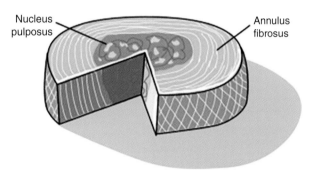

Fig. 1.16 Basic structure of the intervertebral disc. The outer layer, or annulus, is made of layers of collagen and proteoglycan. The inner layer (nucleus pulposus) is a gel-like mixture of water and mucopolysaccharides. (From Waldman S. *Physical Diagnosis of Pain, 2nd ed.* Elsevier; 2021:chap 2, 5-6, Fig. 2.1.)

attached to the anterior margins of the vertebral bodies starting at C1 and extending down to the sacrum and anterior portions of the intervertebral discs. It functions to stabilize the anterior spinal column—notably, during extension.[3]

When using the loss-of-resistance technique while inserting a needle midline, starting dorsally to access the epidural space, one would first encounter the supraspinous ligament, then the interspinous ligament, and the ligamentum flavum. Upon penetration, the ligamentum flavum would result in a loss of resistance in an air-filled or normal saline-filled syringe (Fig. 1.15).[18]

Intervertebral Discs

The first intervertebral disc is found between C2 and C3; the last is between L5 and the sacrum. Disc height and shape varies; cervical and lumbar region discs are wedge shaped and deeper anteriorly than posteriorly, whereas thoracic discs are more uniform in thickness. Lumbar discs are thickest, as they bear a higher proportion of body weight. Disc height decreases with age or due to disc pathology.[16]

The intervertebral discs have two main components: the interior nucleus pulposus and the exterior annulus fibrosus (Fig. 1.16).[19]

The nucleus pulposus is a gel that comprises roughly 50% of the disc. Its position varies based on the vertebral region. In the thoracic region, it is centrally located within the disc; in the cervical and lumbar regions, it is positioned more posteriorly.[20] The annulus fibrosus is made of concentric layers of collagen fibers joined by a proteoglycan gel.

The superior and inferior portion of the vertebral body is a transition region, known as the *vertebral end plate*, where the vertebral body and intervertebral disc interface with each other. The end plate consists of two layers: the first is a thin layer of porous bone that interfaces with the vertebral body, followed by a cartilaginous layer that fuses with the nucleus pulposus of the intervertebral disc (Fig. 1.17).[21] The end plate both prevents the relatively hydrated nucleus pulposus from bulging out of its position and serves a nutritional role, discussed later.[22]

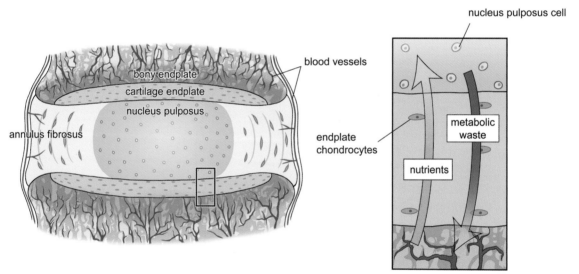

Fig. 1.17 Vertebral end-plate structure and intervertebral disc nutrition. The end plate is composed of a bony layer and a cartilaginous layer. Vertebral capillaries penetrate the bony end plate and terminate at the cartilage end plate, which interfaces with the intervertebral disc. (*Inset*) Small solutes such as glucose and oxygen diffuse in through the cartilage to feed the intervertebral disc. (From Wong J, Sampson SL, Bell-Briones H, et al. Nutrient supply and nucleus pulposus cell function: effects of the transport properties of the cartilage endplate and potential implications for intradiscal biologic therapy. *Osteoarth Cartil.* 2019;27(6):956-964, Fig. 1.)

The adult disc, aside from the outermost annular fibers, is avascular. It relies on diffusion of nutrients and oxygen through blood vessels that surround the outer portions of the annulus fibrosus and from capillary plexuses underneath vertebral end plates, as shown in Fig. 1.17.[21]

Evidence has been found for innervation in the superficial layers of the annulus of the mature disc. It is possible that they have a nociceptive function, which could lead to damaged or degenerated discs as a primary source of back pain.[23,24]

Blood Vessels—Arteries

The spinal cord is supplied by branches from three longitudinal arteries (one anterior spinal artery and two posterior spinal arteries) and several segmental medullary arteries (Fig. 1.18).[25,26]

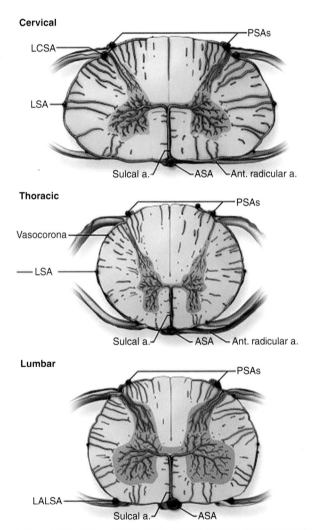

Fig. 1.18 Overview of arterial supply to the spinal cord. The anterior spinal artery (ASA), posterior spinal arteries (PSA), and medullary artery segments are shown. LALSA, lumbosacral anterior spinal arteries; LCSA, lateral cervical spinal arteries; LSA, lateral spinal arterial axis. (Modified from Mauro M, Murphy K, Thomson K, et al. *Image-Guided Interventions*. 3rd ed. Elsevier; 2019:Chap 57, 473-492, Fig. 57.22.)

The anterior longitudinal/spinal artery is formed from branches that exit the two vertebral arteries prior to their convergence to form the basilar artery. From its origin, it then travels down the anterior portion of the spinal cord to the conus medullaris, typically around L1 or L2 (Fig. 1.19). From T3 to T9, the diameter of the anterior longitudinal artery is the smallest. This region of the spinal cord is considered vulnerable to infarct in cases of severe hypotension.[25]

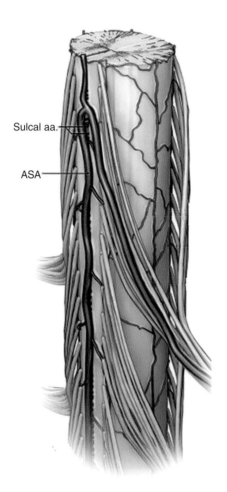

Sulcal aa.

ASA

Fig. 1.19 Course of the anterior spinal artery (ASA), the main arterial supply of the anterior spinal cord. It is formed from branches off the vertebral arteries. It travels along the anterior portion of the spinal cord to the conus medullaris around L1 or L2. Primary and secondary longitudinal chains and their interconnections are depicted as well. (Modified from Mauro M, Murphy K, Thomson K, et al. *Image-Guided Interventions*. 3rd ed. Elsevier; 2019: Chap 57, 473-492, Fig. 57.22.)

The segmental medullary arteries originate from the following. In the cervical region, they originate from the vertebral arteries. In the thoracic region, they originate from the posterior intercostal arteries. In the lumbar region, they originate from various lumbar arteries. Some of these arteries enter the spinal canal by way of the neuroforamina and eventually penetrate the parenchyma of the spinal cord (Fig. 1.20).[1] For the injecting physician, this becomes relevant when performing cervical epidural injections into the intervertebral foramina, as occlusion of the arteries with injectate can cause spinal cord infarction. However, this risk may be partially mitigated with the use of digital subtraction angiography.[27,28]

The vertebral column is supplied by segmental artery branches, also shown in Fig. 1.20. They give rise

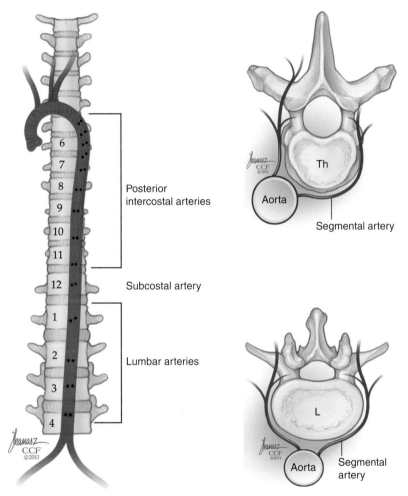

Fig. 1.20 Segmental arteries are part of the arterial supply to the spinal cord and vertebral bodies. (Left) Segmental arteries in the thoracic region arise from the posterior intercostal arteries and in the lumbar region from lumbar arteries. (Right; top and bottom) Segmental arteries entering the spinal cord parenchyma. L, lumbar; Th, thoracic. (From Benzel E. *Spine Surgery: Techniques, Complication Avoidance, and Management.* 5th ed. Vol 1. Elsevier Saunders; 2021:chap 9, 77-97, Fig. 9.24.)

to branches called the *primary periosteal arteries*, which supply the periosteum of vertebral bodies.[1]

Blood Vessels—Veins

The vertebral column is drained by venous plexuses that are exterior and interior to the spinal canal.

The exterior vertebral venous plexus is further divided into anterior and posterior plexuses. The anterior exterior venous plexuses lie in front of the vertebral bodies. The posterior exterior venous plexuses lie over the laminae and spinous and transverse processes, and anastomose with the internal vertebral venous plexus.[29] The interior vertebral venous plexus lies within the spinal canal and spans from the occiput to the coccyx. The veins in this plexus are spread in an arcuate fashion around the spinal canal. The azygos and hemiazygos veins aid in draining the vertebral venous plexuses (Fig. 1.21).[1,29] The interventionalist must be cognizant of these veins, as they can be easy

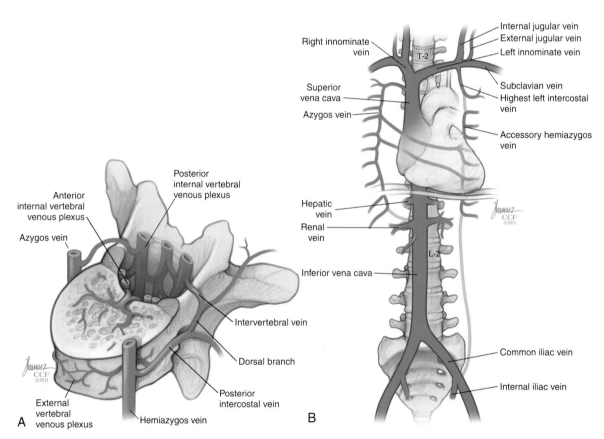

Fig. 1.21 Venous drainage of the spine. The internal and external venous plexuses in relation to the vertebral body. (From Benzel E. *Spine Surgery: Techniques, Complication Avoidance, and Management.* 5th ed. Vol 1. Elsevier Saunders; 2021:chap 9, 77-97, Fig. 9.29.)

sources of bleeding and contribute to post-procedural arachnoiditis, fibrosis of the dura mater or spinal cord, and radiculopathy or myelopathy.

The spinal cord is drained by two median longitudinal veins within the pia mater. One is located anteriorly and one is located posteriorly. These veins drain into the interior vertebral venous plexus, shown in Fig. 1.21.

The Spinal Cord and Nerves

The spinal cord begins immediately below the brain stem, exits the foramen magnum, and ends at the level of the L1 or L2 vertebra, thereafter becoming the cauda equina, a group of nerve roots that innervate the pelvis and lower limbs (Fig. 1.22).[30]

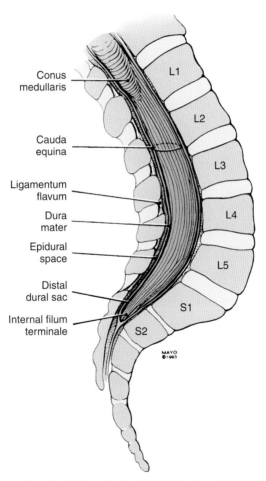

Fig. 1.22 Cauda equina. The spinal cord usually ends at the lower border of the first lumbar vertebral body and then becomes the cauda equina, a group of nerve roots that innervate the pelvis and lower limbs. (From Chestnut D, Wong C, Tsen L, et al. *Chestnut's Obstetric Anesthesia: Principles and Practice.* Elsevier; 2009:chap 12, 238-270, Fig. 12.1.)

The spinal cord is covered first by the adherent pia mater, then the arachnoid mater, then the dura mater more superficially. Between the pia mater and the arachnoid mater is a space known as the *subarachnoid space*. This space contains cerebrospinal fluid (CSF), which bathes the spinal nerves until the space ends at the level of S1/S2, and is known as the *dural sac*. Between the arachnoid mater and the dura mater is a small potential space, known as the *subdural space* (Fig. 1.23).[31] Superficial to the dura mater is the epidural space. Dorsally, it is bordered by the ligamentum flavum and ventrally by the posterior longitudinal ligament. Lateral openings in the epidural space are formed by the intervertebral foramina. The epidural space contains fat and venous plexuses.

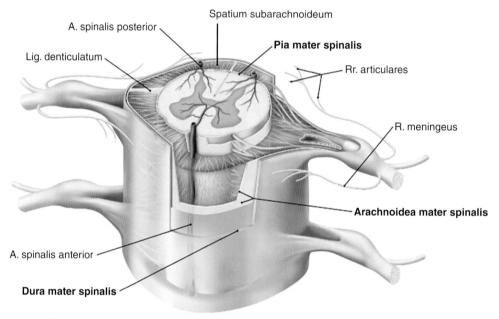

Fig. 1.23 Meninges of the spinal cord; oblique ventral view. The spinal cord is surrounded by the three meninges. Most external is the dura mater, followed by the arachnoid mater. Next, subarachnoid space, which is filled with cerebrospinal fluid (CSF), is encountered. Then, the pia mater, a highly vascularized membrane tightly attached to the surface of the spinal cord, is encountered. Extensions of the pia mater continue laterally on both sides of the spinal cord as denticulate ligaments and serve to stabilize the spinal cord and attach it to the dura mater. (Paulsen, Waschke, Sobotta Atlas of Human Anatomy, 16th Edition 2018 © Elsevier GmbH, Urban & Fischer, Munich.)

Whereas the spinal subarachnoid space is continuous with the intracranial subarachnoid space—hence, the flow of CSF between the brain and spinal cord—the spinal epidural space does not communicate with the intracranial epidural space. The significance of these anatomical relationships is seen when injecting compounds intrathecally (into the subarachnoid space containing CSF), subdurally, or epidurally. Epidural administration of medication requires diffusion through the dura and the arachnoid into the CSF and, thus, has a slower onset of action. Further, when injecting contrast dye, a spread that stops at the superior aspect of C1 denotes epidural injection as opposed to subarachnoid injection (Fig. 1.24).[31]

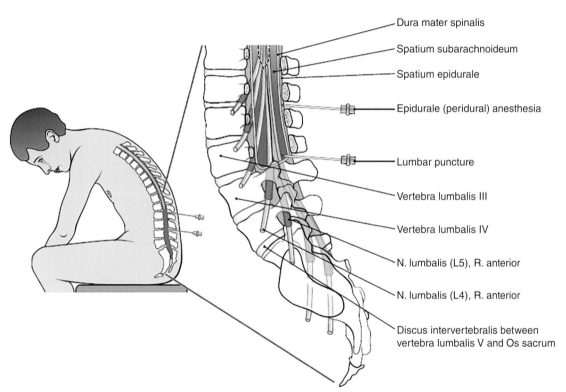

Dura mater spinalis

Spatium subarachnoideum

Spatium epidurale

Epidurale (peridural) anesthesia

Lumbar puncture

Vertebra lumbalis III

Vertebra lumbalis IV

N. lumbalis (L5), R. anterior

N. lumbalis (L4), R. anterior

Discus intervertebralis between vertebra lumbalis V and Os sacrum

Fig. 1.24 Epidural versus intrathecal/spinal needle placement. In epidural needle placement, local adipose tissue restricts the diffusion of the anesthetic into other spinal cord segments. Thus, individual spinal nerves can be selectively anesthetized. In spinal/intrathecal needle placement, the subarachnoid space is accessed. The drug mixes with the cerebrospinal fluid (CSF) but is affected by gravity. Thus, it sinks beneath the injection site (in an upright sitting patient) so that only the nerve branches passing below the injection site will be anesthetized. For lumbar puncture, the tip of the needle lies within the subarachnoid space and CSF can be taken for diagnostic purposes. (Paulsen, Waschke, Sobotta Atlas of Human Anatomy, 16th Edition 2018 © Elsevier GmbH, Urban & Fischer, Munich.)

The spinal cord gives rise to dorsal and ventral nerve roots that join to form a spinal nerve. Each spinal nerve then travels through an intervertebral foramen, after which it bifurcates into a dorsal and ventral ramus as it exits the vertebral column (Fig. 1.25).[32] The ventral nerve roots of the spinal nerve contain axons whose cell bodies are located in the anterior and lateral gray columns of the spinal cord. Ventral nerve root axons contribute somatic efferent nerve fibers to the spinal nerve. The dorsal nerve root of each spinal nerve contains axons whose cell bodies are in the dorsal root ganglia. Dorsal

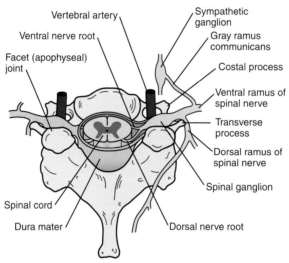

Fig. 1.25 Components of a spinal nerve. The spinal nerve is composed of a dorsal and ventral nerve root. After passing through the intervertebral foramen, it bifurcates into a dorsal and ventral ramus. (From Magee DJ, Manske R. *Orthopedic Physical Assessment*. 7th ed. Elsevier; 2020:chap 1, 1-72, Fig. 1.9.)

nerve root axons are composed of incoming afferent sensory nerve fibers from the periphery that synapse within the dorsal horn of the spinal cord through rootlets, which can number 2 to 15 per level.[6] Dorsal and ventral roots, too, can vary significantly at each spinal level, not only in size and number of roots and dorsal or ventral root ganglia (typically, 1–3 each per level), but also in location of dorsal and ventral root ganglia in relation to their respective foraminae (Fig. 1.26).

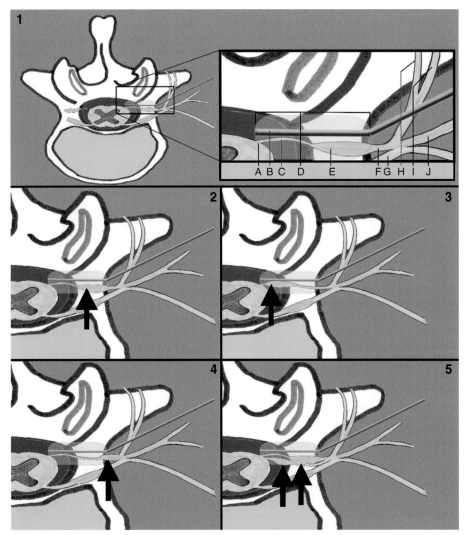

Fig. 1.26 Schematic of variability of dorsal root entry zone complex (DREZC) anatomy in correlation to typical radiofrequency cannula anatomic position. (1) Lumbar vertebra with spinal cord and sensory afferent pathway segments with magnified and labeled view box to the right side. The DREZC is composed of components labelled A, C, E, and F. (A) Dorsal root entry zone (DREZ). (B) Radiofrequency (RF) cannula in typical position, adjacent to the DREZC. (C) Dorsal rootlets (DRLs). The illustration depicts them as one line, but DRLs can vary in number to as many as 15 DRLs per DREZC. (D) The anatomical distribution of the energy wave emitted by the RF cannula. (E) Dorsal root ganglion (DRG). (F) Dorsal root (DR). (G) Ventral root. (H) Medial branch. (I) Intermediate branch. (J) Lateral branch. Panels (2) to (5) show variability in anatomic position and number of DRG relative to the vertebra and RF cannula. *Arrow* depicts DRG. (2) Intraforaminal DRG anatomy. (3) Intraspinal DRG anatomy. (4) Extraforaminal DRG anatomy. (5) DRG biangliar anatomy. (Journal of Pain Research 2021:14 1-12' Originally published by and used with permission from Dove Medical Press Ltd.')

There are 31 pairs of spinal nerves: 8 are cervical, 12 are thoracic, 5 are lumbar, 5 are sacral, and 1 is coccygeal. In relative terms, the cervical nerves exit the vertebral column at the foramen superior to their respective vertebrae (Fig. 1.27). The C3 nerve exits from the C2/C3 foramen located superior to vertebra C3; the C4 nerve exits from the C3/C4 foramen located superior to vertebra C4, until C7 is reached.[19] The C8 nerve then exits from the foramen superior to

the T1 vertebra. After this point, each spinal nerve exits from the foramen inferior to its respective vertebra (Fig. 1.28); spinal nerve T1 exits from the T1/T2 foramen inferior to T1, spinal nerve T2 exits from the T2/T3 foramen inferior to T2, and so on.[33] As there are no intervertebral foramina above C2, the C2 spinal nerve lies atop C2 posterior to the atlantoaxial joint and the C1 spinal nerve lies atop C1 posterior to the atlanto-occipital joint.

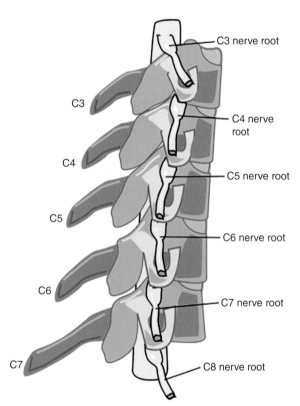

Fig. 1.27 Cervical spinal nerve roots. A cervical nerve exits the vertebral column from the foramen superior to its respective vertebra; for example, the C7 nerve root exits from the foramen superior to the C7 vertebra. (From Waldman S. *Physical Diagnosis of Pain.* Elsevier; 2021: chap 1, 1-4, Fig. 1.6.)

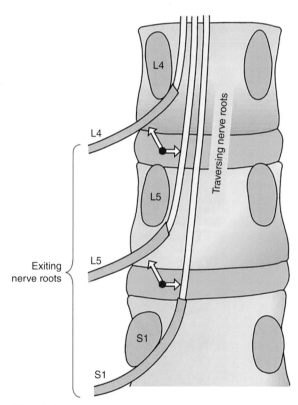

Fig. 1.28 Representation of nerve root exit from the thoracic, lumbar, and sacral vertebral regions. In these regions, a nerve root exits from the foramen below its respective corresponding vertebra. For example, the L5 nerve root exits from the foramen inferior to the L5 vertebra. (Modified from Bogduk N, Tynan W, Wilson AS. The nerve supply to the human lumbar intervertebral discs. *J Anat.* 1981;132(Pt 1):39-56, Fig 2.)

REFERENCES

1. Benzel E, Francis T. *Spine Surgery: Techniques, Complication Avoidance, and Management*. 3rd ed. Philadelphia, PA: Elsevier/Saunders; 2012.
2. Doo AR, Lee J, Yeo GE, et al. The prevalence and clinical significance of transitional vertebrae: a radiologic investigation using whole spine spiral three-dimensional computed tomographic images. *Anesth Pain Med*. 2020;15(1):103-110.
3. Oliver J, Middleditch A. *Funcitonal Anatomy of the Spine*. Jordan Hill, Oxford: Butterworth-Heinemann Ltd; 1991.
4. Auger JD, Frings N, Wu Y, Marty AG, Morgan EF. Trabecular architecture and mechanical heterogeneity effects on vertebral body strength. *Curr Osteoporos Rep*. 2020;18(6):716-726.
5. Witek A, Khalil A, Krishnaney A. Relevant surgical anatomy of the dorsal lumbar spine. In: Manjila S, Mroz T, Steinmetz M, eds. *Lumbar Interbody Fusions*. Philadelphia, PA: 1st ed. Elsevier; 2018:19-25.
6. Tanaka N, Fujimoto Y, An HS, Ikuta Y, Yasuda M. The anatomic relation among the nerve roots, intervertebral foramina, and intervertebral discs of the cervical spine. *Spine (Phila Pa 1976)*. 2000;25(3):286-291.
7. Vo AT, Kim RE, Kirschner JS, Parikh TN, Cohen I, Furman MB. Introduction to fluoroscopic techniques: anatomy, setup, and procedural pearls. In: *Atlas of Image-Guided Spinal Procedures*. Philadelphia, PA: Elsevier; 2018:27-65.
8. Mahadevan V. Anatomy of the vertebral column. *Surgery (Oxford)*. 2018;36(7):327-332.
9. Chakravarthy V, Patel A, Kemp W, Steinmetz M. Surgical treatment of lumbar spondylolisthesis in the elderly. *Neurosurg Clin N Am*. 2019;30(3):341-352.
10. Bazira PJ. Clinically applied anatomy of the vertebral column. *Surgery (Oxford)*. 2021;39(6):315-323.
11. Boreadis AG, Gershon-Cohen J. Luschka joints of the cervical spine. *Radiology*. 1956;66(2):181-187.
12. Silberstein CE. The evolution of degenerative changes in the cervical spine and an investigation into the "Joints of Luschka." *Clin Orthop Relat Res*. 1965;40:184-204.
13. Kayalioglu G. The vertebral column and spinal meninges. In: *The Spinal Cord*. London, UK: Elsevier; 2009:17-36.
14. Shin KH. Percutaneous full-endoscopic interlaminar lumbar spine surgery. In: Kim JS, Lee JH, Ahn Y, eds. *Endoscopic Procedures on the Spine*. Singapore: Springer Nature; 2020:185-209.
15. Rissanen PM. The surgical anatomy and pathology of the supraspinous and interspinous ligaments of the lumbar spine with special reference to ligament ruptures. *Acta Orthop Scand Suppl*. 1960;46:1-100.
16. Benoist M. Natural history of the aging spine. *Eur Spine J*. 2003;12:S86-S89.
17. Ramsey RH. The anatomy of the ligamenta flava. *Clin Orthop Relat Res*. 1966;44:129-140.
18. Waldman S. Cervical epidural block. In: *Atlas of Interventional Pain Management*. Philadelphia, PA: 4th ed. Elsevier; 2015:206-215.
19. Waldman S. Functional anatomy of the cervical intervertebral disc. In: *Physical Diagnosis of Pain*. Philadelphia, PA: 4th ed. Elsevier; 2020:5-6.
20. Koeller W, Meier W, Hartmann F. Biomechanical properties of human intervertebral discs subjected to axial dynamic compression. A comparison of lumbar and thoracic discs. *Spine (Phila Pa 1976)*. 1984;9(7):725-733.
21. Wong J, Sampson SL, Bell-Briones H, et al. Nutrient supply and nucleus pulposus cell function: effects of the transport properties of the cartilage endplate and potential implications for intradiscal biologic therapy. *Osteoarth Cartil*. 2019;27(6):956-964.
22. Sylven B. On the biology of nucleus pulposus. *Acta Orthop Scand*. 1951;20(4):275-279.
23. Wiberg G. Back pain in relation to the nerve supply of the intervertebral disc. *Acta Orthop Scand*. 1949;19(2):211-221.
24. Roofe PG. Innervation of annulus fibrosus and posterior longitudinal ligament: fourth and fifth lumbar level. *Arch Neurol Psychiatry*. 1940;44(1):100.
25. Gailloud P. Arterial anatomy of the spine and spinal cord. In: *Image-Guided Interventions*. Philadelphia, PA: 3rd ed. Elsevier; 2019:473-492.
26. Dommisse GF. The blood supply of the spinal cord. In: *Modern Manual Therapy*. London: Churchill Livingstone; 1986:37-52.
27. Manchikanti L, Candido KD, Singh V, et al. Epidural steroid warning controversy still dogging FDA. *Pain Physician*. 2014;17(4):E451-E474.
28. Scanlon GC, Moeller-Bertram T, Romanowsky SM, Wallace MS. Cervical transforaminal epidural steroid injections: more dangerous than we think? *Spine (Phila Pa 1976)*. 2007;32(11):1249-1256.
29. Batson OV. The vertebral vein system. Caldwell lecture, 1956. *Am J Roentgenol Radium Ther Nucl Med*. 1957;78(2):195-212.
30. Wong CA, Nathan N, Brown DL. Spinal, epidural, and caudal anesthesia: anatomy, physiology, and technique. In: *Chestnut's Obstetric Anesthesia: Principles and Practice*. Philadelphia, PA: Elsevier; 2009:223-245.
31. Paulsen F. Brain and spinal cord. In: *Sobotta Atlas of Anatomy*. Munich, Germany: 16th ed. Elsevier; 2017.
32. Magee D, Manske R. Principles and concepts. In: *Orthopedic Physical Assessment*. St. Louis, MO: 7th ed. Elsevier; 2020.
33. Bogduk N, Tynan W, Wilson AS. The nerve supply to the human lumbar intervertebral discs. *J Anat*. 1981;132(Pt 1):39-56.

Chapter 2

Patient Selection for Vertebral Augmentation

Manuchehr Habibi, Kenneth J. Fiala, and Alaa Abd-Elsayed

Introduction

There is no shortage of health consequences of aging. Osteoporosis, low bone mineral density, and associated vertebral fractures have been a leading cause of diminished quality of life for many people. It was found that the lifetime risk of clinical vertebral fractures at age 50 years is about 15.6% for women and 5% for men.[1] However, only about 33% of people with vertebral fractures develop debilitating symptoms limiting their daily activities.[2] Vertebral augmentation procedures are becoming common for treating osteoporotic vertebral fractures (OVFs) in older patients who have diminished quality of life due to debilitating back pain that limits their physical and daily living activities.[3,4]

Most patients improve with conservative management. However, historically, some patients with unbearable and debilitating pain had to resort to neurosurgery, such as anterior decompression and fusion or posterior instrumentation of the vertebra, which are usually poorly tolerated due to the patient's age and are typically unsuccessful due to the poor quality of bone.[4,5] Consequently, minimally invasive procedures such as vertebroplasty and kyphoplasty, which comprise the vertebral augmentation umbrella, have become a treatment modality of choice.[6] Both percutaneous vertebroplasty and kyphoplasty entail injecting polymethylmethacrylate (PMMA) bone cement into the compressed vertebral body. Kyphoplasty is a modification of vertebroplasty, which involves introducing an inflatable balloon tamp to create a cavity that allows for restoration of the vertebral body height and low-pressure cavity for subsequent cement injection.[7] Kyphoplasty offers a lower risk of cement leakage, reduced incidence of subsequent adjacent fractures, and increases vertebral body height. However, the high cost of this procedure could be a limiting factor.[8] A meta-analysis and systematic review by Wang et al. concluded that both methods are equally effective, yielding similar clinical outcomes.[2] More novel approaches, such as vertebral osteotomy and use of the SpineJack system (Stryker, Kalamazoo, MI), have been developed in recent years that have proved to be promising in decreasing the risk of cement leakage and in improving outcomes. Vertebral osteotomy was found to provide better flexibility in reaching the cracks of the vertebral body where traditional vertebroplasty was unable to do so, reducing the amount of cement used and improving the instability among the adjacent vertebrae.[9] A SpineJack system is a device for mechanical kyphoplasty that resembles a miniature jack with the ability to expand with a large force, in a progressive and controlled manner, in a craniocaudal direction. This allows treatment of fractures that are more chronic—traumatic fractures and primary or secondary bone tumors.[10] Vertebral augmentation has also been increasingly attempted as a palliative treatment of advanced metastatic spine diseases to improve quality of life.[11,12] To optimize these potential benefits of vertebral augmentation, proper patient selection to undergo the procedure is critical.[13]

Relevant Anatomy and Pathophysiology

A human spine consists of a total of 33 vertebrae: 7 cervical, 12 thoracic, 5 lumbar, 5 fused sacral, and 4 fused coccygeal.[14] Each vertebra contains a vertebral body that is typically weakened, deformed, or cracked in patients with osteoporosis. The pain from vertebral fractures is thought to be due to micromotion between the fragments at the fracture site.[15] In some instances, the pain during an acute phase of the fracture can last up to 6 weeks.[16] However, the physiological sequelae, including chronic pain, can remain significantly longer and lead to notable morbidity and mortality. In addition, a patient's tendency toward limited activity or increased bed rest can lead to a vicious pain cycle and increased risk of additional fractures due to further loss of bone mineral density.[17] Inactivity and rest further lead to loss of height and thoracic hyperkyphosis, affecting pulmonary function, causing early satiety, and contributing to mood changes.[17]

Typical conditions that may be treated with vertebral augmentation include osteoporotic vertebral fractures, vertebral hemangiomas, and metastatic lesions.[18]

Candidate Selection

An evaluation of any new patient presenting to a chronic pain clinic begins with focused history, including timing, intensity, and character of the pain. Indication assessment for a patient to undergo a vertebral augmentation procedure should include a history of failure of prior noninterventional options and continuation of intractable pain despite changes in diet; physical therapy; occupational therapy; acupuncture; weight-bearing/impact-loading daily exercises; pharmacological modalities, including antiresorptive agents in conjunction with calcium and vitamin D supplements, and nonopioid and opioid analgesics; and, finally, cessation of smoking.[5] Physical exam findings include tenderness to palpation along the spinous processes without radiation, which typically subsides with sitting or lying supine.[19] Some patients will suffer from psychological manifestations of immobility and the inability to maintain basic activities of daily living, leading to social isolation.[20]

Imaging is essential to candidate selection for vertebral augmentation as it is needed to visualize vertebral damage or degeneration. The fastest, lowest-cost, and most widely available imaging modality to detect spinal fractures remains spinal radiography.[20] However, the best imaging modality to identify and confirm the osteoporotic fractures and differentiate them

from those of neoplastic origin is magnetic resonance imaging (MRI), which is also valuable for distinguishing acute/subacute versus chronic vertebral fractures.[20] Alternatively, a computed tomography (CT) scan with a technetium bone scan can be utilized for patients for whom MRI is contraindicated. A baseline dual-energy X-ray absorptiometry (DEXA) scan is also helpful to assess the risk of future fractures.[17]

Indications for vertebral augmentation are as follows[21]

1. Painful osteoporotic fractures that are resistant to nonoperative management and pharmacological therapy for 3 weeks
2. Pain secondary to bone tumors, such as aggressive hemangioma, giant cell tumor, and bone cysts
3. Pain secondary to extensive osteolysis from multiple myeloma, lymphoma, or metastasis
4. Painful fractures associated with osteonecrosis
5. Traumatic fractures
6. Vertebral body stabilization before open instrumentation surgery

Contraindications to vertebral augmentation include the following[17,21]

1. Fractures improving on medical therapy
2. Highly unstable spine fractures, as in a patient with ankylosing spondylitis or diffuse idiopathic skeletal hyperostosis (DISH)
3. Osteomyelitis or active systemic infection
4. Severe uncorrectable bleeding disorder and coagulopathy
5. Allergy to bone cement or contrast agent
6. Radicular pain, cauda equina syndrome, or myelopathy
7. Fracture of the posterior column, increasing the risk of cement leakage

Complications

Vertebral augmentation procedures have been proven to be a promising alternative to open surgical interventions to treat osteoporotic fractures in the right population. However, as with any procedure, risks such as bleeding, infection, and damage to the surrounding tissues are not negligible. Therefore selecting the correct patients to undergo this procedure is essential to minimize complications. Some case reports exist describing complications such as radiculopathy and paraplegia as a result of cement leakage into the epidural space and neural foramina leading to cord compression,[22] cement pulmonary embolism as a result of liquid PMMA escaping into the venous system,[23] and lumbar arterial injury leading to hemorrhage.[24] In addition, the prevalence of recollapse of the augmented vertebra and adjacent vertebral fracture following the vertebral augmentation has led to exploring risk factors that could be predictive of such complications. Previous studies identified that female gender, low T-score, preoperative intervertebral cleft (IVC), fracture level in the thoracolumbar region, preoperative severe kyphotic deformity, solid lump cement distribution pattern, and higher vertebral height restoration (VHR) were significantly associated with recollapse and adjacent vertebral fracture.[25] With all potential complications in mind, it is essential to weigh the benefits and risks of undergoing a vertebral augmentation procedure. Patients should be selected for these procedures only if the benefits of the procedure outweigh the potential complications. Therefore a thorough assessment of a patient's history, a well-performed physical exam, and proper imaging studies are needed to select patients for vertebral augmentation correctly. This is especially important in older adults for whom the risk of undergoing the procedure may outweigh the benefit.

REFERENCES

1. Johnell O, Kanis J. Epidemiology of osteoporotic fractures. *Osteoporos Int*. 2005;16(2):S3-S7.
2. Wang B, Zhao CP, Song LX, Zhu L. Balloon kyphoplasty versus percutaneous vertebroplasty for osteoporotic vertebral compression fracture: a meta-analysis and systematic review. *J Orthop Surg Res*. 2018;13(1):264.
3. Cooper C. The crippling consequences of fractures and their impact on quality of life. *Am J Med*. 1997;103(2):S12-S19.
4. Hinde K, Maingard J, Hirsch JA, Phan K, Asadi H, Chandra RV. Mortality outcomes of vertebral augmentation (vertebroplasty and/or balloon kyphoplasty) for osteoporotic vertebral compression fractures: a systematic review and meta-analysis. *Radiology*. 2020;295(1):96-103.
5. Dionyssiotis Y. Management of osteoporotic vertebral fractures. *Int J Gen Med*. 2010;3:167-171.
6. Garfin SR, Reilley MA. Minimally invasive treatment of osteoporotic vertebral body compression fractures. *Spine J*. 2002; 2(1):76-80.
7. Hardouin P, Fayada P, Leclet H, Chopin D. Kyphoplasty. *Joint Bone Spine*. 2002;69(3):256-261.
8. Telera S, Raus L, Pipola V, De Iure F, Gasbarrini A. Vertebroplasty and kyphoplasty: an overview. *Vertebral Body Augmentation, Vertebroplasty and Kyphoplasty in Spine Surgery*. 1st ed. Springer; 2021:1-17.
9. He X, Liu Y, Zhang J, et al. An innovative technique for osteoporotic vertebral compression fractures–vertebral osteotome with side-opening cannula. *J Pain Res*. 2018;11:1905-1913.
10. Vanni D, Magliani V, Salini V. Spine jack: evaluation and indications. In: Salini V, Vanni D, eds. *Third Generation Percutaneous Vertebral Augmentation Procedures: Update and Future Perspectives*. New York: Nova Science Publishers; 2015:65-72.
11. Tancioni F, Lorenzetti MA, Navarria P, et al. Percutaneous vertebral augmentation in metastatic disease: state of the art. *J Support Oncol*. 2011;9(1):4-10.
12. Health Quality Ontario. Vertebral augmentation involving vertebroplasty or kyphoplasty for cancer-related vertebral compression fractures: a systematic review. *Ont Health Technol Assess Ser*. 2016;16(11):1-202.
13. Nakamae T, Yamada K, Tsuchida Y, et al. Risk factors for cement loosening after vertebroplasty for osteoporotic vertebral fracture with intravertebral cleft: a retrospective analysis. *Asian Spine J*. 2018;12(5):935-942.
14. Moses KP, Nava PB, Banks JC, Petersen DK. *Atlas of clinical gross anatomy E-book*. 2nd ed. Saunders; 2012.
15. Vanni D, Galzio R, Kazakova A, et al. Third-generation percutaneous vertebral augmentation systems. *J Spine Surg*. 2016; 2(1):13.
16. Suzuki N, Ogikubo O, Hansson T. The course of the acute vertebral body fragility fracture: its effect on pain, disability, and quality of life during 12 months. *Eur Spine J*. 2013;17(10): 1380-1390.
17. Truumees E, Hilibrand A, Vaccaro AR. Percutaneous vertebral augmentation. *Spine J*. 2004;4(2):218-229.
18. Muto M, Muto E, Izzo R, Diano AA, Lavanga A, Di Furia U. Vertebroplasty in the treatment of back pain. *Radiol Med*. 2005;109(3):208-219.
19. Gangi A, Guth S, Imbert JP, Marin H, Dietemann JL. Percutaneous vertebroplasty: indications, technique, and results. *Radiographics*. 2003;23(2):e10.
20. Griffith JF. Identifying osteoporotic vertebral fracture. *Quant Imaging Med Surg*. 2015;5(4):592.
21. Tsoumakidou G, Too CW, Koch G, et al. CIRSE guidelines on percutaneous vertebral augmentation. *Cardiovasc Intervent Radiol*. 2017;40(3):331-342.
22. Lee BJ, Lee SR, Yoo TY. Paraplegia as a complication of percutaneous vertebroplasty with polymethylmethacrylate: a case report. *Spine*. 2002;27(19):E419-E422.
23. Padovani B, Kasriel O, Brunner P, Peretti-Viton P. Pulmonary embolism caused by acrylic cement: a rare complication of percutaneous vertebroplasty. *AJNR Am J Neuroradiol*. 1999; 20(3):375-377.
24. Biafora SJ, Mardjetko SM, Butler JP, McCarthy PL, Gleason TF. Arterial injury following percutaneous vertebral augmentation: a case report. *Spine*. 2006;31(3):E84-E87.
25. Yu W, De Liang ZY, Qiu T, Ye L, Huang X, Jiang X. Risk factors for recollapse of the augmented vertebrae after percutaneous vertebroplasty for osteoporotic fractures with intravertebral vacuum cleft. *Medicine*. 2017;96(2):e5675.

Chapter 3

Perioperative Care for Vertebral Augmentation

Alaa Abd-Elsayed and Ahish Chitneni

Preoperative Care

Various procedures are used today for vertebral augmentation, including percutaneous vertebroplasty, balloon augmentation, vertebral osteotomy augmentation, and kyphoplasty—for example, the SpineJack system (Stryker, Michigan, USA). Preoperative, intraoperative, and postoperative care for each procedure remains mainly similar but considerations for each procedure must be made. Prior to the procedure, a patient must meet the indications for undergoing a vertebral augmentation. Current guidelines state that a patient may be eligible for vertebral augmentation if the patient has severe limitation of function due to pain or hospitalization due to a vertebral compression fracture (VCF), a history of VCFs, and physical examination shows tenderness with palpation or percussion over the spinous processes that is further confirmed by imaging showing VCF.[1] Contraindications for the procedure include patients with an underlying infection, osteomyelitis, or other surgical site infections.[1] An additional contraindication is that patients with osteoporotic compression fracture may benefit from medication management as the use of kyphoplasty and vertebroplasty in acute osteoporotic compression fractures may have limited benefit per current research.[2] Another relative contraindication for a kyphoplasty may be a VCF with a posterior cortical breach.[3] Prior to the procedure, various labs and diagnostic tests are ordered for operative clearance: complete blood count (CBC), basic metabolic panel (BMP), prothrombin time and international normalized ratio (PT/INR), and review of all X-ray and magnetic resonance imaging (MRI). One reason for the lab workup includes ruling out reduced kidney function to avoid exacerbating the condition due to contrast-induced nephropathy.[4] Prior to the procedure, anticoagulation and antiplatelet medications are put on hold per guidelines for spinal anesthesia.[5] In many cases, aspirin and nonsteroidal anti-inflammatory drugs (NSAIDs) are also held for 7 days and 2 to 3 days prior to the procedure, respectively.[5]

Intraoperative Care

In general, patients typically undergo a vertebral augmentation procedure in an outpatient surgical center. Patients typically receive local or mild sedation. However, in some situations, general anesthesia may be advised. The type of sedation administered typically will correlate to the procedure being done, number of compression fractures, and the length of the procedure.[5] The treatment of a single-level VCF generally has a total procedure time of less than 1 hour and local anesthesia is typically used. In cases in which multilevel VCF treatment is being done, general anesthesia may be a consideration.[5] Several complications can occur during and after both kyphoplasty and vertebroplasty procedures. Some complications include spinal cord compression, embolism, infection, and radicular pain.[6] Local cement leakage is another complication with both vertebroplasty and kyphoplasty, with vertebroplasty showing a higher percentage of patients with local cement leakage.[7]

Postoperative Care

In general, postoperative care for vertebral augmentation includes the application of an adhesive bandage at the puncture site. After completion of the procedure, patients are typically discharged home from the post-anesthesia care unit or recovery room several hours after the procedure. During their stay in the recovery room, various signs indicating allergic reactions are closely monitored and appropriately treated.[5] One of the most important parts of postoperative management after vertebral augmentation is the treatment of postoperative pain. The use of ice at the surgical site is recommended for pain relief and discomfort. In addition, a short course of opioids is the first-line treatment for post-procedural pain, with the goal of tapering those medications and transitioning to acetaminophen and NSAIDs for pain relief.[5]

REFERENCES

1. Clerk-Lamalice O, Beall DP, Ong K, Lorio MP. ISASS Policy 2018—Vertebral augmentation: coverage indications, limitations, and/or medical necessity. *Int J Spine Surg.* 2019;13(1):1-10.

2. Ebeling PR, Akesson K, Bauer DC, et al. The efficacy and safety of vertebral augmentation: a second ASBMR Task Force report. *J Bone Miner Res.* 2019;34(1):3-21.

3. Molloy S, Sewell MD, Platinum J, et al. Is balloon kyphoplasty safe and effective for cancer-related vertebral compression fractures with posterior vertebral body wall defects? *J Surg Oncol.* 2016;113(7):835-842.

4. Dydyk AM, Das JM. Vertebral augmentation. In: *StatPearls* [Internet]. Treasure Island, FL: StatPearls Publishing; 2022.

5. Luginbühl M. Percutaneous vertebroplasty, kyphoplasty and lordoplasty: implications for the anesthesiologist. *Curr Opin Anaesthesiol.* 2008;21(4):504-513.

6. Saracen A, Kotwica Z. Complications of percutaneous vertebroplasty: an analysis of 1100 procedures performed in 616 patients [published correction appears in *Medicine (Baltimore)*. 2016;95(31):e5074]. *Medicine (Baltimore)*. 2016;95(24):e3850.

7. Taylor RS, Taylor RJ, Fritzell P. Balloon kyphoplasty and vertebroplasty for vertebral compression fractures: a comparative systematic review of efficacy and safety. *Spine (Phila Pa 1976)*. 2006;31(23):2747-2755.

Vertebroplasty/Kyphoplasty: Transpedicular Approach

Lucas Vannoy and Keth Pride

Introduction

Percutaneous vertebroplasty is an image-guided procedure for the injection of bone cement into the vertebral body. The benefits of vertebroplasty include bone strengthening and potential decompression of spinal nerves with increased mobility to improve quality of life.[1]

Vertebroplasty is indicated for patients with osteoporotic vertebral body collapse and osteolytic metastases or myeloma who have severe pain refractory to conservative pain medication management. Vertebral body compression fractures are estimated to occur approximately 700,000 times each year.[2] Vertebroplasty is recommended and performed by some providers for immediate pain relief and decompression shortly after vertebral body collapse. However, standard medical treatment includes analgesics, rest, and external bracing. Typical improvement occurs over 4 to 6 weeks and approximately two-thirds of patients will improve with only conservative management. The most common indication for vertebroplasty is treatment of acute vertebral body compression fracture for patients who do not respond to conservative medical therapy after 6 weeks.[3]

Vertebroplasty and kyphoplasty are performed similarly. However, a kyphoplasty enables the option for a biopsy to be taken or a drill to be utilized to create a path for a balloon tamponade system. In contrast to vertebroplasty, kyphoplasty is usually performed via a bipedicular approach.

Indications

- Treatment of painful vertebral compression fractures secondary to osteoporosis refractory to conservative management
- Treatment of painful vertebral compression fractures secondary to metastatic neoplasia refractory to conservative management
- Patients are best identified by looking for the appropriate symptoms and signs, which include:
  - Fractures that occur with little or no trauma
  - Deep pain with sudden onset
  - Midline location of pain
  - Exacerbation of pain with axial loading
  - Pain refractory to conservative management
  - Pain exacerbated by motion (especially twisting)
  - Point tenderness over fractured vertebra

Vertebroplasty is not indicated for patients with mild to moderate pain responding to medical management. The American Society for Bone and Mineral Research advises to avoid vertebroplasty for patients with acute osteoporotic vertebral fractures.

Contraindications

- Active systemic infection
- Uncorrectable bleeding diathesis
- Insufficient cardiopulmonary health to safely undergo the necessary anesthesia
- Myelopathy secondary to epidural tumoral extension
- Allergy to bone cement

Perioperative Considerations

All patients should not eat or drink for at least 6 hours prior to the procedure. The required level of sedation may vary from local anesthesia and moderate sedation to general anesthesia. That said, having the patient awake is desirable because it allows real-time feedback that can inform the practitioner of potential intraoperative complications or neurological dysfunction. In all cases, sedation and monitoring are performed by anesthesiologists, nurse anesthetists, or certified nursing personnel. For anticoagulation status and recommendations regarding antibiotic prophylaxis, refer to previously published guidelines.

Trajectory Safety Considerations

ANTEROPOSTERIOR VIEW SAFETY CONSIDERATIONS

- Avoid spinal cord and thecal sac by staying lateral to medial border of the pedicle (Fig. 4.1).[4]
- Avoid nerve roots and spinal nerves by staying within the pedicular borders (Fig. 4.2).

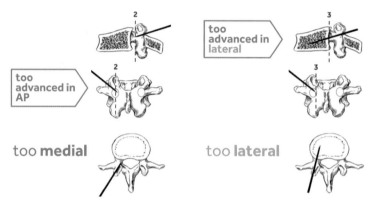

Fig. 4.1 Proper needle trajectory pathway from lateral view (*top*), anteroposterior view (*middle*), and axial view (*bottom*) with alignment correction recommendations. (Courtesy Medtronic.)

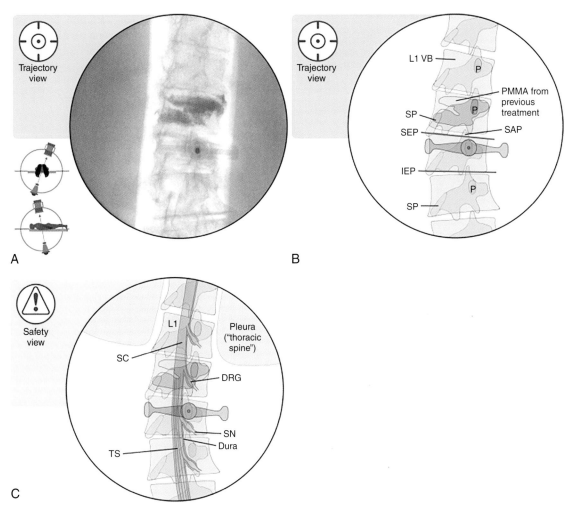

Fig. 4.2 (A) Fluoroscopic image of a trajectory view with the affected L3 vertebral body "squared off" with the pedicle in line with the vertebral body. Cannulate the vertebral body in the trajectory view. (B) Radiopaque structures. (C) Radiolucent structures. (From Furman MB, Frey ME. Sacral insufficiency fracture repair/sacroplasty. In: Furman MB, Berkwits, Cohen I, et al., eds. *Atlas of Image-Guided Spinal Procedure.* 2nd ed. Elsevier; 2018:337–348; Fig. 19.1.)

LATERAL VIEW SAFETY CONSIDERATIONS

- Once through the pedicle, view the cannula tip in the lateral view, which should be seen at the posterior vertebral body wall (see Figs. 4.1 and 4.3).

- Penetrating the anterior vertebral body could damage the aorta/inferior vena cava.
- Improper trajectory could penetrate the inferior wall of the pedicle resulting in possible spinal nerve damage.

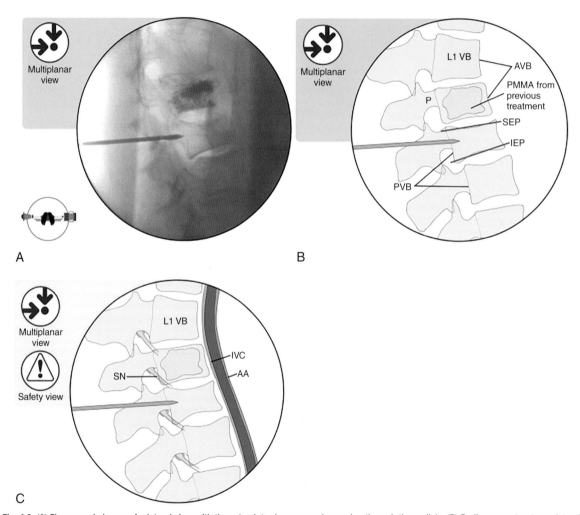

A B C

Fig. 4.3 (A) Fluoroscopic image of a lateral view with the osteo introducer cannula passing through the pedicle. (B) Radiopaque structures, lateral view. (C) Radiolucent structures, lateral view. (From Furman MB. Sacral insufficiency fracture repair/sacroplasty. In: Furman MB, Berkwits, Cohen I, et al., eds. *Atlas of Image-Guided Spinal Procedure.* 2nd ed. Elsevier; 2018:337–348; Fig. 19.3.)

Step-by-Step Procedural Description

PEDICULAR ADVANCEMENT

1. Confirm the vertebral level with the anteroposterior view.
2. Craniocaudally tilt the C-arm to level the inferior end plate of the targeted vertebral body (see Fig. 4.2).
3. Tilt the C-arm ipsilateral oblique, usually 10 to 20 degrees, with the pedicle appearing as a rounded clock face, so that the pedicle is superimposed within the outline of the vertebral body (Figs. 4.4 and 4.5).
4. The cannula entry point is determined by the vertebral fracture location. Most fractures occur along the superior end plate; therefore, the superior lateral quadrant of the pedicle should be the entry point. For biconclave and planar fractures, enter at the middle of the pedicle. For inferior end-plate fractures, entry should be in the inferior lateral quadrant (see Fig. 4.4).

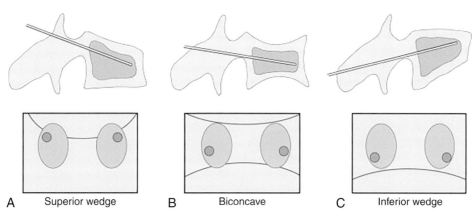

A Superior wedge B Biconcave C Inferior wedge

Fig. 4.4 Pedicle entry points and trajectories. (A) Superior end-plate compressions should be approached by directing the cannula toward the inferior end plate in the lateral view. (B) Biconcave fracture cannulation should take place in the center of the vertebral body. (C) Inferior compression fractures will require more of a cephalad cannula trajectory. (From Furman MB. Sacral insufficiency fracture repair/sacroplasty. In: Furman MB, Berkwits, Cohen I, et al., eds. *Atlas of Image-Guided Spinal Procedure.* 2nd ed. Elsevier; 2018:337–348; Fig. 19.11.)

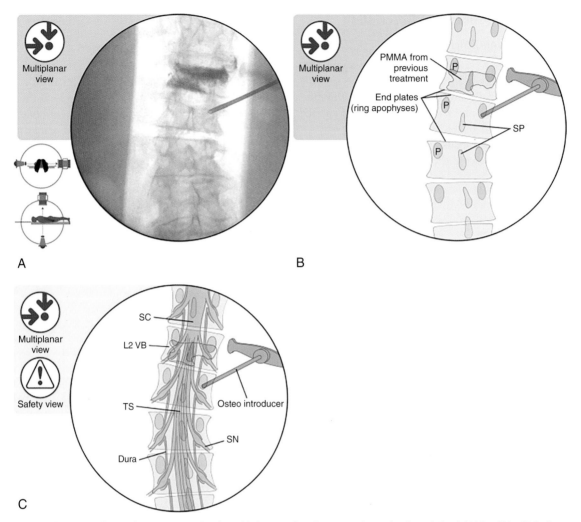

Fig. 4.5 (A) Fluoroscopic image of an anteroposterior view with the osteo introducer cannula passing through the right L3 pedicle. (B) Radiopaque structures, anteroposterior view. (C) Radiolucent structures, anteroposterior view. (From Furman MB. Sacral insufficiency fracture repair/sacroplasty. In: Furman MB, Berkwits, Cohen I, et al., eds. *Atlas of Image-Guided Spinal Procedure*. 2nd ed. Elsevier; 2018:337–348; Fig. 19.2.)

5. Local anesthetic should be administered in the superficial and overlying tissues.
6. Make the skin incision.
7. Insert osteo-introducer device or bone needle and align with proper entry site as described in Step 4 via fluoroscopy (see Figs. 4.4, 4.6, and 4.7).
8. Gently tap the bone needle to create a starting hole; slowly advance with tapping or manual pressure (Fig 4.8).

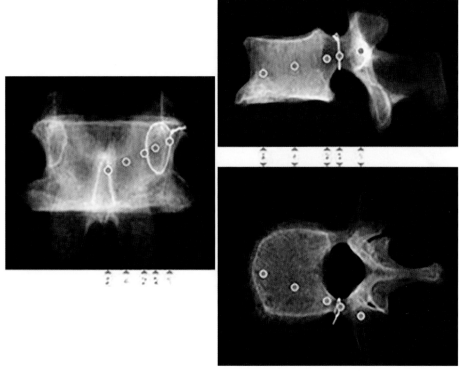

Fig. 4.6 Proper needle trajectory pathway from the anteroposterior view (*top left*), lateral view (*top right*), and axial view (*bottom*). (Courtesy Medtronic.)

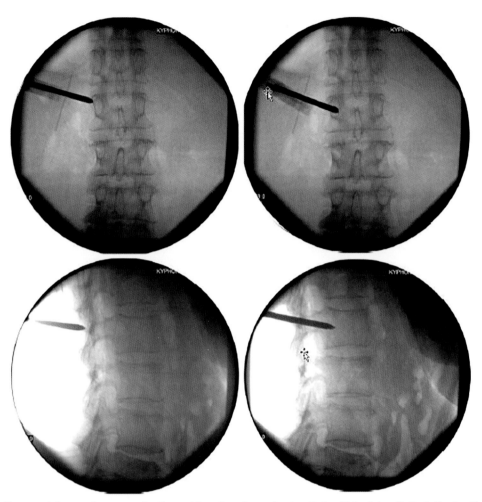

Fig. 4.7 Fluoroscopic images of proper needle alignment from the anteroposter view (*top*) and lateral view (*bottom*). (Courtesy Medtronic.)

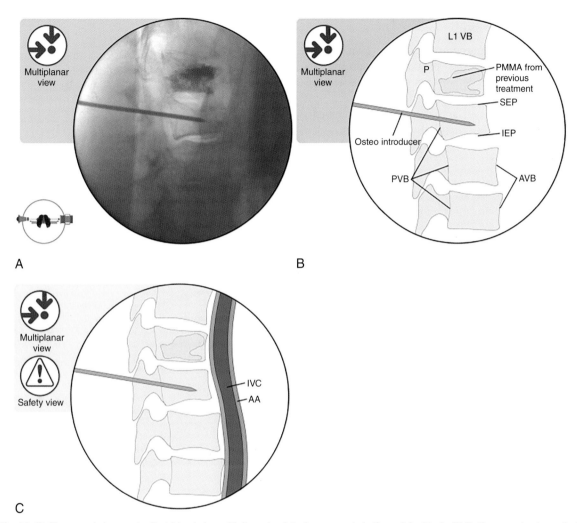

Fig. 4.8 (A) Fluoroscopic image of a final lateral view with the osteo introducer cannula in the vertebral body. (B) Radiopaque structures, final lateral view. (C) Radiolucent structures, final lateral view. (Source: Furman MB. Atlas of Image-Guided Spinal Procedure. 2nd ed. Elsevier; 2018: chap 19, Fig. 19.5, 337–348.)

Bone Cement Injection

1. Begin live fluoroscopy (typically, lateral view). The view should include anterior/posterior structures to demonstrate any inadvertent cement extravasation (anterior can advance into the great vessels and cause cement pulmonary embolism). Intermittently stop to also check the anteroposterior view to evaluate for lateral extravasation to the foramen (Figs. 4.9 to 4.11).

2. Inject a half turn (0.5 mL) at a time. If completing kyphoplasty, the volume injected should roughly equal the amount of contrast injected into a balloon tamponade (Fig. 4.13).

3. Stop the injection once contrast is seen *toward* or *past* the midline (see Fig. 4.13).

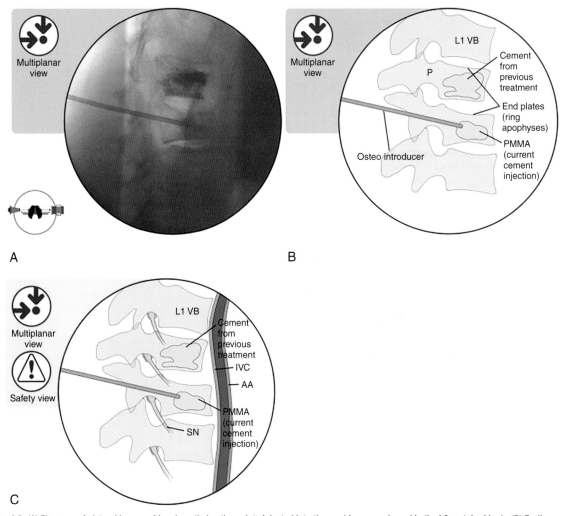

Fig. 4.9 (A) Fluoroscopic lateral image with polymethylmethacrylate injected into the working cannula and in the L3 vertebral body. (B) Radiopaque structures, lateral view. (C) Radiolucent structures, lateral view. (From Furman MB. Sacral insufficiency fracture repair/sacroplasty. In: Furman MB, Berkwits, Cohen I, et al., eds. *Atlas of Image-Guided Spinal Procedure.* 2nd ed. Elsevier; 2018:337–348; Fig. 19.7.)

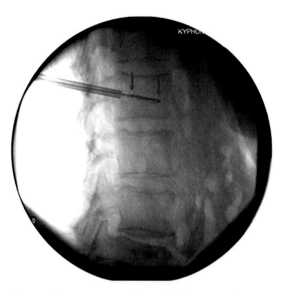

Fig. 4.10. Fluoroscopic lateral image of bone cement cannula insertion along proper alignment (*arrows*). (Courtesy Medtronic.)

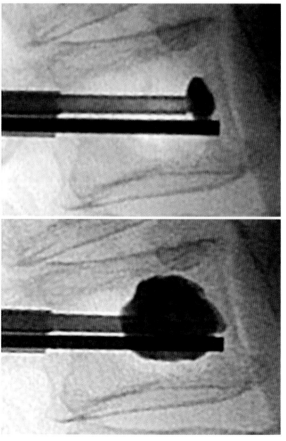

Fig. 4.11 Fluoroscopic lateral image of bone cement progressively being injected into vertebral body. (Courtesy Medtronic.)

KYPHOPLASTY TECHNIQUE PEARLS

- Begin bone drill use after osteo introducer tip is placed at the anterior to posterior cortex line of the vertebral body (Fig. 4.12).
- Inflate bone tamponade in 0.25- or 0.5-mL increments to reduce fracture risk (Fig. 4.13).

- Do not increase total volume beyond 4 mL with 10-mm or 15-mm bone tamponade or 6 mL with 20-mm tamponade.
- Stop inflation if there is cortical wall contact, balloon reaches maximum volume, or pressure reaches 400 psi.

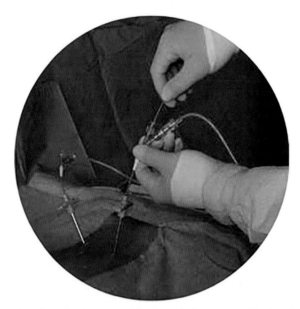

Fig. 4.12 External view of vertebroplasty cannula hardware for bone cement injection. (Courtesy Medtronic.)

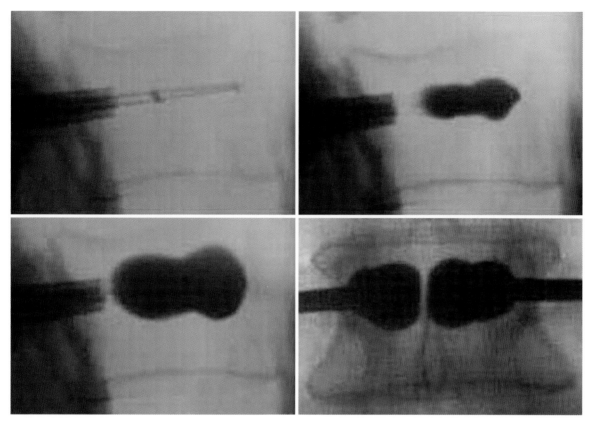

Fig. 4.13 Fluoroscopic images in lateral view of unilateral bone cement cannula insertion (*top left*) and subsequent single balloon inflation (*top right*). Lateal view showing even distribution of bone cement in vertebral body (*bottom left*). Fluoroscopic image in anteroposterior view showing bilateral kyphoplasty balloon inflation (*bottom right*). (Courtesy Medtronic.)

Intraoperative Complications

A severe osteoporotic spine presents an increased risk for intraoperative complications of spine interventions. Infectious complications such as osteomyelitis are possible but extremely rare. A small retrospective cohort study demonstrates a significantly greater risk of subsequent vertebral fracture following this procedure. New fracture is also a possibility where risk factors for new compression fracture include low bone mineral density (BMD), intradiscal cement leakage, and vertebral height restoration.[5] Extravasation of cement has been reported in 11% to 73% of procedures, but this is not clinically relevant unless it occurs in the spinal canal or neural foraminae, which is rare.[5] Finally, pulmonary cement emboli were reported in 5% to 23% via chest radiography, none of which caused clinical symptoms.[5]

Postoperative Considerations

Bone cement setting time is typically less than 10 minutes and the procedure is complete after hemostasis is achieved.[3] After that, patients should be kept supine for 2 hours. A postprocedural neurological exam should then be completed to compare with a baseline exam. If there is no change and the patient can ambulate, the patient can then be discharged home. We do not recommend routine bracing. Patient activity should be kept to a minimum for 1 to 2 days. Significant pain improvement is typically reported within 2 to 7 days.[3]

In a review of 30 studies with more than 2000 patients with osteoporotic vertebral fracture treated with vertebroplasty, major complications that may require surgical intervention occurred in 0.9% of patients, and no deaths were reported.[3] Complications that have been described include bleeding, infection, transient radiculopathy, spinal stenosis, and rare allergic reaction to bone cement. In a review of 69 clinical studies, cement extravasation has been reported in 41% of cases, with 96% being asymptomatic.[3]

REFERENCES

1. Liu JC, Bendok BR Chapter 61. In: Benzon HT, Raja SN, Molloy RE, Liu SS, Fishman SM, eds. Essentials of Pain Medicine and Regional Anesthesia. Elsevier; 2005:494–515. 2nd ed.
2. Reeves R, Ante WA, Frey ME, Furman MB. Vertebral Augmentation (Vertebroplasty/Kyphoplasty): Transpedicular Approach. In: Furman MB, Berkwits L, Cohen I, eds, et al. Atlas of Image-Guided Spinal Procedure. Vertebral Augmentation (Vertebroplasty/Kyphoplasty): Transpedicular Approach. Elsevier; 2018:337–348. 2nd ed.
3. Jay B, Ahn SH. Vertebroplasty. *Semin Intervent Radiol.* 2013; 30(3):297–306.
4. Medtronic. *Kyphon Balloon Kyphoplasty Physician Training* [PowerPoint Slides]. 2021.
5. Rosen HN, Walega DR. Osteoporotic Thoracolumbar Vertebral Compression Fractures: Clinical Manifestations and Treatment. UpToDate. https://www.uptodate.com/contents/osteoporotic-thoracolumbar-vertebral-compression-fractures-clinical-manifestations-and-treatment?search=Rosen%20HN,%20Walega%20DR.%20Osteoporotic%20Thoracolumbar%20Vertebral%20Compression%20Fractures:%20Clinical%20Manifestations%20and%20Treatment.%20UpToDate;%206%2F9%2F2021&source=search_result&selectedTitle=1~150&usage_type=default&display_rank=1. Accessed 6/9/2021.
6. Benzon HT, Rathmell JP, Wu CL, et al., eds. Minimally invasive Procedures for Vertebral Compression Fractures. In: Practical Pain Management. Elsevier; 2014:922–932. 5th. ed.

Chapter 5

Balloon Augmentation

David J. Mazur-Hart, Nasser K. Yaghi, and Ahmed M. Raslan

Introduction

Back pain remains one of the most common complaints seen by primary care and pain treatment providers. Lifetime prevalence has been reported to be as high as 84%.[1] Roughly 11% of the population is disabled due to low back pain. Back pain has many etiologies and can be difficult to treat. On the other hand, some forms of back pain can be readily diagnosed and can be treated successfully with proven therapeutic interventions. One proven intervention for some types of back pain is vertebral body augmentation, which includes both vertebroplasty and kyphoplasty. This chapter will focus specifically on kyphoplasty.

Kyphoplasty differs slightly from vertebroplasty. A report of treatment with vertebroplasty was first published in 1987.[2] It involves filling a vertebral body with an acrylic cement, polymethyl methacrylate (PMMA). PMMA solidifies within the vertebral body to prevent further damage by providing structural support to the vertebral body. There is also a theory that the reaction of the cement solidifying within the vertebral body may damage local intrinsic pain fibers.[3] This, in turn, shortens the duration of pain experienced and prevents worsening kyphosis. Kyphoplasty was developed as an evolution of vertebroplasty and was first performed in 1998.[4] Kyphoplasty differs in that it involves inflating a balloon inside the vertebral body to create a cavity for the PMMA (Fig. 5.1). The balloon allows for height restoration and improvement in focal kyphosis prior to filling.

The rest of the chapter will focus on specific aspects of kyphoplasty. It will cover indications, contraindications, diagnostic workup, and the procedure. Kyphoplasty can be safely performed as an outpatient procedure by a well-trained proceduralist.

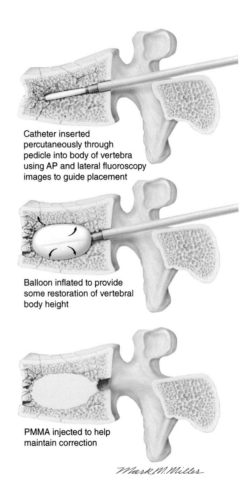

Catheter inserted percutaneously through pedicle into body of vertebra using AP and lateral fluoroscopy images to guide placement

Balloon inflated to provide some restoration of vertebral body height

PMMA injected to help maintain correction

Fig. 5.1 Illustration of kyphoplasty being performed on lumbar compression fracture. (From Greene W. *Netter's Orthopaedics.* In: Metabolic Bone Disease and Osteonecrosis. Saunders; 2006: 39, Image ID: 8127.)

Indications

1. Severe pain or progressive collapse of a vertebral body in the setting of osteoporosis or osteopenia
   - *Osteoporotic compression fracture:* A review found that physical disability, general health,

and pain relief were improved with vertebroplasty and kyphoplasty compared with medical management within 3 months of intervention.[5] Another review found improvements in pain, functionality, vertebral height, and kyphotic angle at least 3 years post-procedure comparing kyphoplasty with medical management.[6] Another review comparing vertebroplasty, kyphoplasty, and nonsurgical management found that vertebroplasty and kyphoplasty provided significantly more pain reduction over nonsurgical management with no difference in pain reduction between vertebroplasty and kyphoplasty.[7] They also found that subsequent fractures occurred more frequently in the nonsurgical group compared with surgical groups. Additionally, there was greater kyphosis reduction and less cement extravasation in patients in kyphoplasty groups over vertebroplasty groups. Another review comparing vertebroplasty and kyphoplasty found no significant difference in pain reduction or disability scores. However, they did find lower odds of new fractures, less extraosseous cement leakage, and greater reduction in kyphotic angle with kyphoplasty.[8] A randomized controlled trial found a statistically significant improvement in mean SF-36 Pain Catastrophizing Scale (PCS) score between the kyphoplasty group and nonsurgical group.[9]

- *Osteonecrosis (Kümmell disease):* A randomized controlled trial compared kyphoplasty with a bone-filling mesh container and found that both improved visual analog scale (VAS) scores, Oswestry Disability Index (ODI) scores, and Cobb angles.[10] Another trial comparing kyphoplasty with vertebroplasty found both a decrease in VAS scores and ODI scores with no significant difference between techniques.[11]

2. Severe pain or progressive collapse of a vertebral body in the setting of neoplasm
   - *Vertebral metastasis:* A review found that patients with spine metastasis treated with kyphoplasty had better scores for pain, disability, quality of life, and functional status.[12] Another review found that pain scores decreased, often within 48 hours of the procedure, and analgesic use decreased along with noted improvement in mean pain-related disability scores.[13] Finally, a randomized controlled trial found a statistically significant improvement in Roland-Morris disability questionnaire (RDQ) scores between kyphoplasty and control groups.[14]
   - *Multiple myeloma:* A systematic review found that vertebroplasty and kyphoplasty were equally effective at lowering pain scores in patients with multiple myeloma.[15]
   - *Vertebral hemangioma:* A small case series and review of the literature found kyphoplasty to be successful in the management of painful spine hemangiomas.[16]

3. Severe pain or progressive collapse of a vertebral body in the setting of trauma
   - There are small studies that indicate improved pain and earlier mobilization without bracing after kyphoplasty for non-osteoporotic traumatic fractures.[17-19]

Contraindications

- Active infection at the target vertebral level
- Sepsis, blood-borne illness, systemic infection
- Burst fracture or disrupted posterior vertebral body wall
- Neurological deficit
- Spinal instability
- Nonpainful fracture, healed fracture
- Pain responding to conservative therapy

Complications

- PMMA leak
  - Central canal
  - Neural foramen
  - Disc space
  - Soft tissue
  - Venous, with possible pulmonary embolism[20]
- Radiculopathy, possibly from thermodynamics of cement hardening[3]
- Hemo- or pneumothorax by anterior vertebral wall puncture
- New iatrogenic fracture: pedicle, transverse process, rib
- Hematoma from needle tract
- Future adjacent level fracture

Workup

- Standing upright X-ray (XR) anteroposterior (AP) and lateral views to evaluate height loss and angulation
- Computed tomography (CT) of the spine to evaluate posterior wall
- Magnetic resonance imaging to evaluate for acute fracture (short T1 inversion recovery [STIR])
- Dual-energy X-ray absorptiometry (DEXA) scan to evaluate for osteoporosis/osteopenia
- Bone scintigraphy in setting of multiple pathological levels because the most active level can correlate with the most successful intervention level

Procedure

1. *Setup.* Various vendors provide the supplies for balloon augmentation. We will describe a generic approach to the procedure. The procedure requires fluoroscopy, which can be performed in an operating room, angiography suite, or procedure room. Some providers prefer using two C-arm machines in a "nested" technique to avoid switching one machine between AP and lateral images. The O-arm intraoperative CT scanner can also be used for rapid AP and lateral images using the scout XR function without performing a full CT. The procedure can be performed under general anesthesia, sedation, or local anesthesia.

2. *Positioning.* The patient is positioned prone on a radiolucent table. For most thoracic and lumbar vertebral levels, the arms should be positioned with the shoulders abducted 90 degrees and elbows flexed 90 degrees in the "Superman" position and padded to prevent any brachial plexus or peripheral nerve palsies.

3. *Localization.* The vertebral level is marked on the skin using lateral radiographs with a radio-opaque object. The radiographs must be exactly perpendicular to the intended level. We align the spinous process directly midway between pedicles on AP XR with a single radiodensity of the superior and inferior end plates of the target level. This will yield a clear view down the column of the pedicles (Fig. 5.2). On the lateral XR, we overlie the pedicles and create a single radiodensity of the superior and inferior end plates of the target

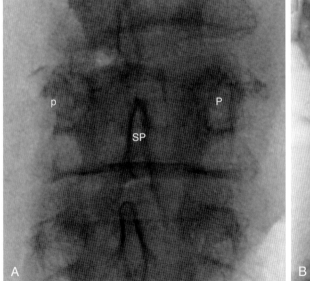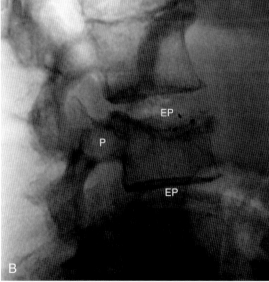

Fig. 5.2 Safe kyphoplasty begins with true orthogonal views on anteroposterior (AP) and lateral fluoroscopic views. (A) AP view showing "owl eyes" appearance of round pedicles (P) as the eyes and spinous process (SP) as the beak. (B) Lateral view showing single radiodensity of superior and inferior end plates (EP).

level (see Fig. 5.2). Obtaining the appropriate XR views in the AP and lateral orientations is one of the most critical steps to performing this procedure effectively and safely. We mark out bilateral stab incisions roughly 3 cm lateral to the midline at the target level using a lateral XR. If needed, AP radiographs can be used for additional confirmation.

4. *Preparation.* If hair is present, it may be minimally clipped. The area is prepared in a sterile manner and the patient and fluoroscopy machine are draped in a sterile manner. A timeout is performed. Radiographs with a radio-opaque object are again performed to ensure appropriate levels and entry points (Fig. 5.3). If needed, the planned incision is remeasured and marked as the skin can move during cleaning and draping. Local anesthetic is injected, including the dermis through the paraspinal musculature, ensuring that no amount is given intravascularly or intrathecally.

5. *Incision.* A stab incision is made, often with a #11 scalpel blade, into the subcutaneous tissues. A Jamshidi (BD, Franklin Lakes, NJ) needle is passed through the soft tissues under AP radiographic guidance until resting on cortical bone at the pedicle entry point, which is the

lateral aspect of the pedicle at the midpoint of the pedicle's vertical height (Fig. 5.4A). Lateral radiographs may be obtained for confirmation to ensure alignment (Fig. 5.4B). This entry point will slightly vary based on the anatomy of the pedicle at the targeted vertebral level. The

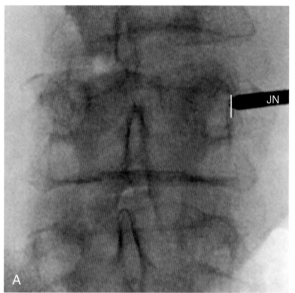

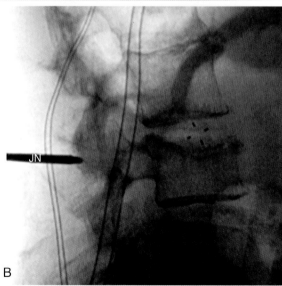

Fig. 5.3 Confirmation lateral radiograph with radio-opaque object (O) to ensure appropriate level and trajectory.

Fig. 5.4 (A) Anteroposterior and (B) lateral radiographs showing appropriate entry point into pedicle with Jamshidi needle (JN). The *white vertical line* outlines the lateral board of the pedicle.

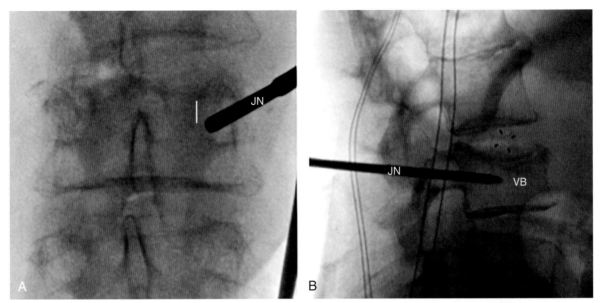

Fig. 5.5 (A) Anteroposterior and (B) lateral radiographs depicting safe trajectory through the pedicle and into the vertebral body (VB). The trajectory of the Jamshidi needle (JN) should aim to transverse from the lateral to medial pedicle wall as the needle is advanced. The *white vertical line* outlines the medial board of the pedicle.

Jamshidi needle is tapped with a mallet to hold its position in cortical bone.

6. *Pedicle Entry.* The mallet is then used to advance the Jamshidi needle through the pedicle and into the vertebral body using AP radiographs to ensure alignment within the pedicle walls (Fig. 5.5). The trajectory of the needle should aim to transverse from the lateral to medial pedicle wall as the needle is advanced 2 cm, which is roughly the length of thoracolumbar pedicles. The Jamshidi needle must not be medial to the pedicle, as this puts the spinal cord at risk for iatrogenic injury (see Fig. 5.5). Likewise, the Jamshidi needle must not be lateral to the pedicle to prevent cement extravasation into an unintended location. The C-arm is moved into a lateral position to confirm appropriate positioning of the Jamshidi needle into the vertebral body. The tip of the needle should allow for the passage of the balloon into the anterior half of the vertebral body.

7. *Balloon Preparation.* The inner stylet of the Jamshidi needle is removed. A hand twist drill is advanced to core out a space for the insertion of the balloon (Fig. 5.6). The balloon tubing is

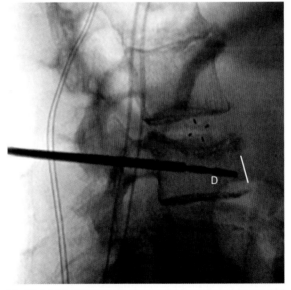

Fig. 5.6 Lateral radiograph showing that the inner stylet of the Jamshidi needle has been removed and an inner hand twist drill (D) has been placed. This cores out a small area for the balloon. Care is taken not to pierce the anterior cortical bone of the vertebral body. The *white oblique line* outlines the most anterior cortical bone of the vertebral body.

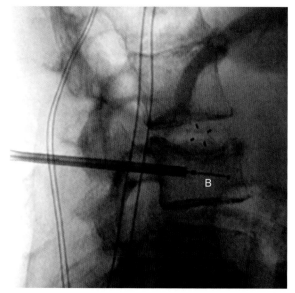

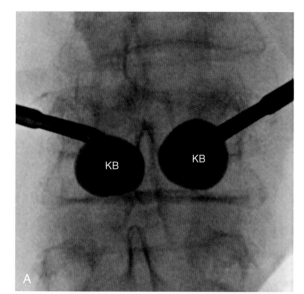

Fig. 5.7 Lateral radiograph with the balloon (B) showing radio-opaque identifiers (*small black dots*) at the proximal and distal ends of the balloon are observed outside the cannula of the Jamshidi needle.

filled with radio-opaque contrast to allow visualization on radiographs. The balloon is passed down the inner cannula and advanced out the end of the needle into the anterior half of the vertebral body.

8. *Balloon Insertion.* The balloon will have radio-opaque markers that need to be visualized outside the cannula to allow for full inflation of the balloon (Fig. 5.7).

9. *Balloon Insufflation.* The balloon is inflated slowly under monitored pressure and intermittent fluoroscopy to create a cavity to increase vertebra height, improve kyphosis, and create a space for the cement. Different vendors will recommend varying upper pressure limits. This upper pressure limit is designed to decrease the chance of fracturing cortical bone that would allow a pathway for cement leakage. AP and lateral radiographs are used to ensure appropriate insufflation, which is midline and contained by cortical bone circumferentially (Fig. 5.8).

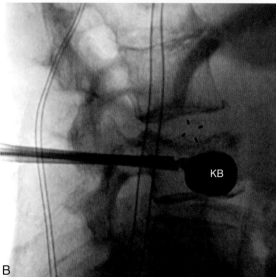

Fig. 5.8 (A) Anteroposterior and (B) lateral radiographs depicting inflation of the kyphoplasty balloons (KB) filled with radio-opaque contrast. The superior end plate has been expanded cranially.

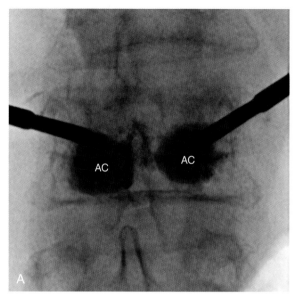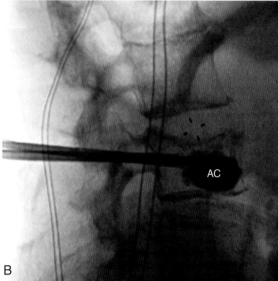

Fig. 5.9 (A) Anteroposterior and (B) lateral radiographs showing that the acrylic cement (AC) has filled the balloon cavities. Care is taken to avoid cement extravasation.

10. *Cement Augmentation.* The balloon is deflated rapidly and removed. The cavity is then filled with PMMA (Fig. 5.9). Vendors will supply an optimal fill volume, along with instructions on how to prepare the PMMA, which needs to be discussed in advance to ensure an appropriate timing window for PMMA use. The cement is inserted slowly down the cannula and into the vertebral body while carefully observing for leakage in any direction under both AP and lateral radiographs.

11. *Closure.* Once satisfied with deployment of the cement, the remaining portions of the Jamshidi needles are removed and final radiographs are obtained. The small skin incisions can be cleaned and closed with absorbable suture or simply a bandage.

Conclusion

Balloon augmentation by kyphoplasty is a safe and proven intervention in providing relief for targeted pathologies of back pain. It can be performed in an operating room or procedure room in the outpatient setting. Further developments in kyphoplasty are directed at considerations for a unilateral versus bilateral approach. The idea is to decrease intervention time and radiation exposure with the hope of obtaining similar clinical outcomes. Results have been controversial. Recent systematic reviews suggest similar clinical scores, radiological outcomes, and quality of life with a unilateral kyphoplasty, with the advantages of shorter procedure times, smaller cement volumes, lower cement leak risk, lower radiation dose, and decreased cost.[21-24]

REFERENCES

1. Balagué F, Mannion AF, Pellisé F, Cedraschi C. Non-specific low back pain. *Lancet.* 2012;379(9814):482-491.
2. Galibert P, Deramond H, Rosat P, Le Gars D. [Preliminary note on the treatment of vertebral angioma by percutaneous acrylic vertebroplasty]. *Neurochirurgie.* 1987;33(2):166-168.
3. Greenberg MS. *Handbook of Neurosurgery.* Thieme; 2016.
4. Beall DP. *Vertebral Augmentation: The Comprehensive Guide to Vertebroplasty, Kyphoplasty, and Implant Augmentation.* Georg Thieme Verlag; 2020.
5. McGirt MJ, Parker SL, Wolinsky JP, Witham TF, Bydon A, Gokaslan ZL. Vertebroplasty and kyphoplasty for the treatment of vertebral compression fractures: an evidenced-based review of the literature. *Spine J.* 2009;9(6):501-508.

6. Taylor RS, Fritzell P, Taylor RJ. Balloon kyphoplasty in the management of vertebral compression fractures: an updated systematic review and meta-analysis. *Eur Spine J.* 2007;16(8):1085-1100.

7. Papanastassiou ID, Phillips FM, Van Meirhaeghe J, et al. Comparing effects of kyphoplasty, vertebroplasty, and non-surgical management in a systematic review of randomized and non-randomized controlled studies. *Eur Spine J.* 2012;21(9):1826-1843.

8. Gu CN, Brinjikji W, Evans AJ, Murad MH, Kallmes DF. Outcomes of vertebroplasty compared with kyphoplasty: a systematic review and meta-analysis. *J Neurointerv Surg.* 2016;8(6):636-642.

9. Wardlaw D, Cummings SR, Van Meirhaeghe J, et al. Efficacy and safety of balloon kyphoplasty compared with non-surgical care for vertebral compression fracture (FREE): a randomised controlled trial. *Lancet.* 2009;373(9668):1016-1024.

10. Duan ZK, Zou JF, He XL, Huang CD, He CJ. Bone-filling mesh container versus percutaneous kyphoplasty in treating Kümmell's disease. *Arch Osteoporos.* 2019;14(1):109.

11. Chang JZ, Bei MJ, Shu DP, Sun CJ, Chen JB, Xiao YP. Comparison of the clinical outcomes of percutaneous vertebroplasty vs. kyphoplasty for the treatment of osteoporotic Kümmell's disease: a prospective cohort study. *BMC Musculoskelet Disord.* 2020;21(1):238.

12. Astur N, Avanzi O. Balloon kyphoplasty in the treatment of neoplastic spine lesions: a systematic review. *Global Spine J.* 2019;9(3):348-356.

13. Health Quality Ontario. Vertebral augmentation involving vertebroplasty or kyphoplasty for cancer-related vertebral compression fractures: a systematic review. *Ont Health Technol Assess Ser.* 2016;16(11):1-202.

14. Berenson J, Pflugmacher R, Jarzem P, et al. Balloon kyphoplasty versus non-surgical fracture management for treatment of painful vertebral body compression fractures in patients with cancer: a multicentre, randomised controlled trial. *Lancet Oncol.* 2011;12(3):225-235.

15. Khan OA, Brinjikji W, Kallmes DF. Vertebral augmentation in patients with multiple myeloma: a pooled analysis of published case series. *AJNR Am J Neuroradiol.* 2014;35(1):207-210.

16. Jones JO, Bruel BM, Vattam SR. Management of painful vertebral hemangiomas with kyphoplasty: a report of two cases and a literature review. *Pain Physician.* 2009;12(4):E297-E303.

17. Hartmann F, Gercek E, Leiner L, Rommens PM. Kyphoplasty as an alternative treatment of traumatic thoracolumbar burst fractures Magerl type A3. *Injury.* 2012;43(4):409-415.

18. Zaryanov AV, Park DK, Khalil JG, Baker KC, Fischgrund JS. Cement augmentation in vertebral burst fractures. *Neurosurg Focus.* 2014;37(1):E5.

19. Grelat M, Madkouri R, Comby PO, Fahed E, Lemogne B, Thouant P. Mid-term clinical and radiological outcomes after kyphoplasty in the treatment of thoracolumbar traumatic vertebral compression fractures. *World Neurosurg.* 2018;115:e386-e392.

20. Choe DH, Marom EM, Ahrar K, Truong MT, Madewell JE. Pulmonary embolism of polymethyl methacrylate during percutaneous vertebroplasty and kyphoplasty. *AJR Am J Roentgenol.* 2004;183(4):1097-1102.

21. Xiang GH, Tong MJ, Lou C, Zhu SP, Guo WJ, Ke CR. The role of unilateral balloon kyphoplasty for the treatment of patients with OVCFS: a systematic review and meta-analysis. *Pain Physician.* 2018;21(3):209-218.

22. Zhiyong C, Yun T, Hui F, Zhongwei Y, Zhaorui L. Unilateral versus bilateral balloon kyphoplasty for osteoporotic vertebral compression fractures: a systematic review of overlapping meta-analyses. *Pain Physician.* 2019;22(1):15-28.

23. Sun H, Lu PP, Liu YJ, et al. Can unilateral kyphoplasty replace bilateral kyphoplasty in treatment of osteoporotic vertebral compression fractures? A systematic review and meta-analysis. *Pain Physician.* 2016;19(8):551-563.

24. Tan G, Li F, Zhou D, Cai X, Huang Y, Liu F. Unilateral versus bilateral percutaneous balloon kyphoplasty for osteoporotic vertebral compression fractures: a systematic review of overlapping meta-analyses. *Medicine (Baltimore).* 2018;97(33):e11968.

Chapter 6

Vertebral Augmentation With Osteotome

Clayton Busch, Nasir Hussain, and Alaa Abd-Elsayed

Introduction

The incidence of vertebral compression fracture is estimated at 800,000 per year in the United States, and they often result in hospitalization.[1] Osteoporotic compression fractures affect 30% to 50% of people older than 50 years.[2] Additionally, the vertebral column is a common site for painful bone metastases and multiple myeloma, which results in vertebral fractures on presentation in up to 70% of patients.[3,4] Diagnosis and treatment of compression fractures is important, as these injuries can lead to chronic back pain, pulmonary dysfunction, recurrent falls, severe compromise of activities of daily life, reduced quality of life, and greater health care utilization.[1,5,6] These fractures are also a chief factor of morbidity in cancer patients.[3] Furthermore, vertebral fractures are an underappreciated cause of morbidity and mortality among the elderly.[7]

Treatment for vertebral compression fractures begins with medical management with bracing, oral pain medications, and rest.[8] If conservative therapy fails after 3 weeks (and preferably before 6 weeks), the patient should be referred to be evaluated for interventional therapy (i.e., vertebral augmentation).[9,10]

Vertebroplasty was first performed to treat an aggressive cervical hemangioma; other indications surfaced in the literature of the late 1980s.[11] A variation in the technique referred to as "kyphoplasty" was described in 2001 by Garfin and Lieberman in which balloons were used in an attempt to restore vertebral height prior to introduction of cement.[12,13] As surgical treatments evolve, further techniques and technologies continue to be introduced to this familiar procedure, such as the recent method of vertebral augmentation with osteotome.

Vertebral Augmentation With Osteotome

A cadaveric study using a prototype curved osteotome for vertebral augmentation was published in 2002.[14] Clinical studies were further described in the late 2000s.[15,16] While Zhong and colleagues report clinical application with a curved osteotome for vertebral augmentation since 2013,[17] the curved osteotome differs in methodology from vertebroplasty in that there is more significant cavity creation prior to cement administration. It also differs from balloon kyphoplasty in that the pre-cement maneuver allows greater control of the shape, size, and direction of the cavity created for the cement.

The advantage of cavity creation addresses the issue of cement leakage. Nontarget cement leakage is the most common complication of vertebral augmentation procedures, which can result in pulmonary embolism or nerve damange.[18] In vertebroplasty, higher pressures build as cement is injected to the fractured vertebrae. Kyphoplasty offers a lower-pressure alternative by creating a cavity with the balloon first.[9] Vertebral augmentation with osteotome offers a more refined approach to cavity creation prior to cement injection. A curved or maneuverable osteotome can be guided to selected portions of the vertebrae. This preserves cancellous bone that otherwise would have been destroyed by a balloon kyphoplasty.[19] Advantages of a vertebral augmentation osteotome include amenability to the unipedicular approach, directional control of the osteotome, a side hole for cement delivery that prevents inadvertent administration of cement to soft tissues upon withdrawal of the cannula, and preservation of the native cancellous bone matrix[15,16,19] (Figs. 6.1 and 6.2).

The benefits of using an osteotome have also been reported in the literature. In one head-to-head study, unilateral curved osteotome utilization was compared with more traditional bilateral vertebroplasty and was

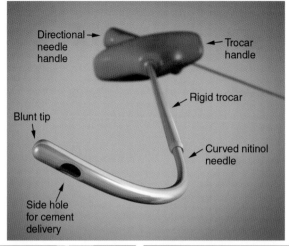

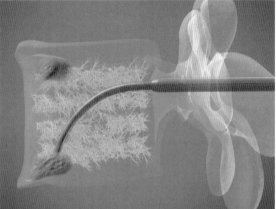
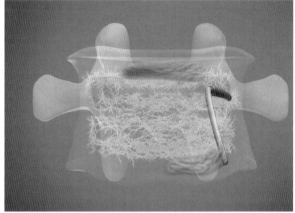

Fig. 6.1 A curved vertebral augmentation osteotome is pictured as it would be inserted through a rigid trocar. These images depict how a curved osteotome can be used to target a specific location within the vertebrae. (From Brook AL, Miller TS, Fast A, Nolan T, Farinhas J, Shifteh K. Vertebral augmentation with a flexible curved needle: preliminary results in 17 consecutive patients. *J Vasc Interv Radiol.* 2008;19(12):1785-1789.)

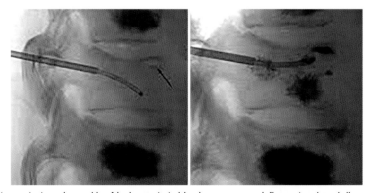

Fig. 6.2 The precision that an osteotome is capable of is demonstrated in vivo on a young inflammatory bowel disease patient with osteoporosis secondary to long-term steroid use. A contralateral subendplate cleft is successfully targeted and filled with cement. (From Hunt CH, Kallmes DF, Thielen KR. A unilateral vertebroplasty approach using a curved injection cannula for directed, site-specific vertebral body filling. *J Vasc Interv Radiol.* 2009;20(4):553-555.)

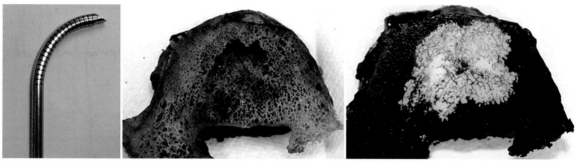

Fig. 6.3 A navigational osteotome achieves significant interdigitation into cancellous bone after cement injection. (From Murphy K. Radiofrequency kyphoplasty: a novel approach to minimally invasive to treatment of vertebral compression fractures. In: Yue JJ, Guyer R, Johnson JP, et al., eds. *The Comprehensive Treatment of the Aging Spine: Minimally Invasive and Advanced Techniques.* Saunders/Elsevier; 2011:248-252, Fig. 40.2.)

found to have significantly lower operation time, lower number of fluoroscopic images taken, and lower cement leakage rate. Importantly, both techniques demonstrated similar improvement in pain and disability indices at 1 year after the procedure.[17] Vertebral augmentation with osteotome, like kyphoplasty, achieves reductions in kyphotic deformity.[17,19,20] However, there are still a limited amount of comparisons between balloon kyphoplasty and osteotome vertebral augmentation for kyphotic deformity.

Cancellous bone preservation is an area of interest for the future of vertebral augmentation procedures. Specifically, there has been interest in incorporating calcium and other related biological substances into cements that would eventually merge into native bone. Unfortunately, this cannot be done with typical balloon-based systems due to the absence of Haversian canal systems.[18] Cements and other technologies amenable to osteotomes leave this field ripe for innovation. Operator-controlled curving of the osteotome and radiofrequency technology for more controlled cement hardening are two such examples.[19,21] Significant interdigitation of the cement injection is noted using these technologies[22] (Fig. 6.3).

Patient Selection and Evaluation

The success of any procedure begins with proper patient selection. Indications for vertebral augmentation with osteotome are similar to that of vertebroplasty or balloon kyphoplasty. Vertebral compression fractures that are nonresponsive to medical management (i.e.,

worsening pain symptoms or function) within 3 to 6 weeks should be further evaluated.[9,10] However, positive results from performing vertebroplasty or kyphoplasty have been reported even when used as far as 2 years out from the initial injury.[8] A neurological examination (motor abnormalities, sensory abnormalities, existing radiculopathies) should be performed, and routine lab work and coagulation studies should be obtained. If fractures are secondary to malignancy, an appropriate workup should be undertaken. Imaging with X-rays, computed tomography scans, and magnetic resonance imaging may also be beneficial.[8] Bone marrow or end-plate edema are positive prognostic indicators for vertebral augmentation.[8]

INDICATIONS[11]

- Osteoporotic vertebral compression fractures not responding to conservative management
- Bony metastases to the vertebrae with significant osteolysis (including multiple myeloma)
- Kummel disease
- Symptomatic vertebral hemangiomas
- Need for anterior stabilization prior to surgical operation to be performed on the posterior spine
- Traumatic fracture within 10 days with kyphotic angle > 15 degrees

Procedural Technique

Vertebroplasty/kyphoplasty has been described in detail in previous chapters. Briefly, the procedure is performed via a transpedicular approach with the patient placed in a prone position and sedated using monitored general anesthesia. However, local anesthesia can also be used. First, an introducer is advanced through a transpedicular approach under fluoroscopic guidance. The introducer is advanced to the posterior fourth of the vertebral body. An inner puncture needle is then removed and subsequently replaced with an orientation device with the curved injection cannula and osteotome. The curved osteotome and cannula can then be advanced to the contralateral side (or region of interest) by the proceduralist under fluoroscopic guidance. When the site is reached by the osteotome, the inner osteotome is withdrawn with the outer cannula remaining in place. Cement is subsequently injected point by point while the cannula is withdrawn.[17]

Contraindications

Absolute contraindications to vertebral augmentation include asymptomatic vertebral compression fractures, unstable spine fractures, diffuse idiopathic skeletal hyperostosis, ankylosing spondylitis, osteomyelitis, discitis, active infection, severe uncorrectable coagulopathy, or allergy to bone cement or opacification agents.[10] Relative contraindications include radicular pain, tumor extension to the vertebral canal or cord compression, fracture of the posterior column, sclerotic metastasis, and diffuse metastasis.[10] Additional contraindications include vertebral metastases with spinal canal involvement, pregnancy, severe cardiorespiratory disease, and local infection at the procedure site.[11]

Conclusion

Vertebral augmentation with osteotome is a newer technique than vertebroplasty and balloon kyphoplasty. It has been less thoroughly investigated than traditional vertebroplasty and balloon kyphoplasty techniques; however, the data available are promising. The benefits of reduced patient and operator radiation exposure, shorter procedure times, and similar long-term patient outcomes suggest promise with these approaches and technologies. Furthermore, the tools that can work well with the osteotome and the osteotome's amenability to new cement technologies show promise in the treatment of vertebral compression fractures in the future.

REFERENCES

1. Wood KB, Li W, Lebl DR, Lebl DS, Ploumis A. Management of thoracolumbar spine fractures. *Spine J.* 2014;14(1):145-164.
2. Ballane G, Cauley JA, Luckey MM, El-Hajj Fuleihan G. Worldwide prevalence and incidence of osteoporotic vertebral fractures. *Osteoporos Int.* 2017;28(5):1531-1542.
3. Mansoorinasab M, Abdolhoseinpour H. A review and update of vertebral fractures due to metastatic tumors of various sites to the spine: percutaneous vertebroplasty. *Interv Med Appl Sci.* 2018;10(1):1-6.
4. Lieberman I, Reinhardt MK. Vertebroplasty and kyphoplasty for osteolytic vertebral collapse. *Clin Orthop Relat Res.* 2003;(suppl 415):S176-S186.
5. Beall DP, Olan WJ, Kakad P, Li Q, Hornberger J. Economic analysis of Kiva VCF treatment system compared to balloon kyphoplasty using randomized Kiva Safety and Effectiveness Trial (KAST) data. *Pain Physician.* 2015;18(3):E299-E306.
6. Ross PD. Clinical consequences of vertebral fractures. *Am J Med.* 1997;103(2A):30S-42S; discussion, 42S-43S.
7. Papaioannou A, Watts NB, Kendler DL, Yuen CK, Adachi JD, Ferko N. Diagnosis and management of vertebral fractures in elderly adults. *Am J Med.* 2002;113(3):220-228.
8. Fessler RD, Lebow RL, O'Toole JE, Fessler RG, Eichholz KM. Percutaneous vertebral augmentation: vertebroplasty and kyphoplasty. In: Scuderi GR, Tria AJ, eds. *Minimally Invasive Surgery in Orthopedics.* 2nd ed. Cham: Springer; 2016:1129-1144.
9. Long Y, Yi W, Yang D. Advances in vertebral augmentation systems for osteoporotic vertebral compression fractures. *Pain Res Manag.* 2020;2020:3947368.
10. Tsoumakidou G, Too CW, Koch G, et al. CIRSE Guidelines on percutaneous vertebral augmentation. *Cardiovasc Intervent Radiol.* 2017;40(3):331-342.
11. Filippiadis DK, Marcia S, Masala S, Deschamps F, Kelekis A. Percutaneous vertebroplasty and kyphoplasty: current status, new developments and old controversies. *Cardiovasc Intervent Radiol.* 2017;40(12):1815-1823.
12. Garfin SR, Yuan HA, Reiley MA. New technologies in spine: kyphoplasty and vertebroplasty for the treatment of painful osteoporotic compression fractures. *Spine (Phila Pa 1976).* 2001;26(14):1511-1515.
13. Lieberman IH, Dudeney S, Reinhardt MK, Bell G. Initial outcome and efficacy of "kyphoplasty" in the treatment of painful osteoporotic vertebral compression fractures. *Spine (Phila Pa 1976).* 2001;26(14):1631-1638.
14. Murphy KJ, Lin DD, Khan AA, Gailloud P. Multilevel vertebroplasty via a single pedicular approach using a curved 13-gauge needle: technical note. *Can Assoc Radiol J.* 2002;53(5):293-295.
15. Brook AL, Miller TS, Fast A, Nolan T, Farinhas J, Shifteh K. Vertebral augmentation with a flexible curved needle: preliminary results in 17 consecutive patients. *J Vasc Interv Radiol.* 2008;19(12):1785-1789.
16. Hunt CH, Kallmes DF, Thielen KR. A unilateral vertebroplasty approach using a curved injection cannula for directed, site-specific vertebral body filling. *J Vasc Interv Radiol.* 2009;20(4):553-555.
17. Zhong R, Liu J, Wang R, et al. Unilateral curved versus bipedicular vertebroplasty in the treatment of osteoporotic vertebral compression fractures. *BMC Surg.* 2019;19(1):193.
18. Hargunani R, Le Corroller T, Khashoggi K, Murphy KJ, Munk PL. Percutaneous vertebral augmentation: the status of vertebroplasty and current controversies. *Semin Musculoskelet Radiol.* 2011;15(2):117-124.

19. Dalton BE, Kohm AC, Miller LE, Block JE, Poser RD. Radiofrequency-targeted vertebral augmentation versus traditional balloon kyphoplasty: radiographic and morphologic outcomes of an ex vivo biomechanical pilot study. *Clin Interv Aging.* 2012;7:525-531.

20. He X, Liu Y, Zhang J, et al. An innovative technique for osteoporotic vertebral compression fractures—vertebral osteotome with side-opening cannula. *J Pain Res.* 2018;11:1905-1913.

21. Hegazy R, El-Mowafi H, Hadhood M, Hannout Y, Allam Y, Silbermann J. The outcome of radiofrequency kyphoplasty in the treatment of vertebral compression fractures in osteoporotic patients. *Asian Spine J.* 2019;13(3):459-467.

22. Murphy K. Radiofrequency kyphoplasty: a novel approach to minimally invasive treatment of vertebral compression fractures. In: Yue JJ, Guyer RD, Johnson JP, Khoo LT, Hochschuler SH, eds. *The Comprehensive Treatment of the Aging Spine: Minimally Invasive and Advanced Techniques.* Saunders/Elsevier; 2011:248-252.

Chapter 7

Vertebral Augmentation Using Expandable Intravertebral Implants

Pooja Chopra, Kailash Pendem, Genevieve Marshall, and Navdeep S. Jassal

Introduction

Osteoporotic vertebral compression fracture (OVCF) is one of the most common manifestations of osteoporosis. OVCFs occur in approximately 20% of individuals over 70 years of age.[1] The fractures can cause persistent pain and result in an overall decrease in quality of life. Treatment goals of OVCF include reduction of pain and stabilization of the vertebrae. Conservative treatment includes rest, activity modification, analgesics, and bracing. However, conservative treatment can be ineffective for some patients and surgical intervention can prove to be helpful in those with significant vertebral instability or neurological compromise.[2]

Vertebroplasty and kyphoplasty are the standard methods for minimally invasive treatment of vertebral compression fractures. Vertebroplasty involves the percutaneous injection of polymethylmethacrylate (PMMA) bone cement directly into the fractured vertebral body to stabilize the OVCF. Balloon kyphoplasty (BKP) addresses the kyphotic deformity as well as the fracture pain. The procedure involves insertion of an inflatable bone tamp to elevate end plates. This restores the vertebral body back to its original height and creates a cavity to be filled with a bone cement.[3] There is potential for intraprocedural loss of vertebral height as the balloon deflates.[4] Several clinical and biomechanical studies have shown that there is a height loss after deploying the balloons.[4,5]

Newer intravertebral reduction devices improve anatomical restoration of the end plates of the vertebral body. The SpineJack (SJ) system (Stryker Corporation, Kalamazoo, MI) is an expandable metal implant (titanium alloy) mounted on an expander, two of which are inserted bilaterally into the vertebral body and simultaneously expanded. The SJ was designed to restore vertebral shape and stabilize the fractured vertebra. The expandable implant is inserted before the injection of the bone cement in order to prevent secondary loss of vertebral body height, which can be observed in BKP. In biomechanical studies, the device has been shown to be superior to BKP in terms of sagittal height restoration and height maintenance.[4,5] Furthermore, the SAKOS trial was a prospective, multicenter, randomized study that successfully demonstrated noninferiority of the SJ system to BKP with an excellent risk–benefit profile over 12 months. Adjacent-level fractures are the most commonly cited procedure-related adverse event in various single-center studies of SJ outcomes. SAKOS demonstrated radiographic superiority of the SJ over BKP with freedom from adjacent-level fractures and minor superiority for midline vertebral body height restoration at 6 and 12 months.[6]

Anatomy

OVCF often occur at the midthoracic (T7–T8) spine and the thoracolumbar junction (T12–L1). The 12 thoracic vertebrae are intermediate in size between the cervical and lumbar vertebrae (Fig. 7.1). The thoracic spine maintains a slight kyphosis and each vertebral body articulates with the rib cage. The thoracolumbar junction is susceptible to injury and instability because the spinal column progresses from the stable thoracic spine to the more mobile lumbar spine at this level.[7]

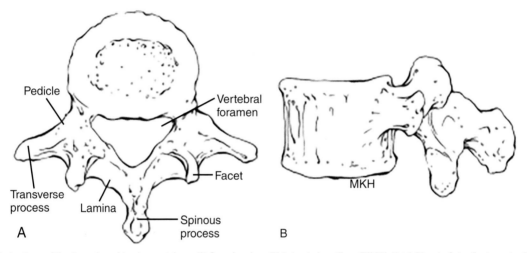

Fig. 7.1 Anatomy of the thoracic and lumbar vertebrae. **(A)** Superior view. **(B)** Lateral view. (From Eiff PM, Hatch RL, eds. Spine Fractures. In: *Fracture Management for Primary Care and Emergency Medicine*. 4th ed. Elsevier; 2019; Fig. 10.15.)

Diagnosis

Initial imaging for an OVCF should include anteroposterior (AP), lateral, and oblique views of the entire thoracolumbar spine because many patients have fractures at more than one level.[8] Anterior and posterior vertebral body heights are compared to determine severity of vertebral fractures and are staged as follows.[9]

- Grade 1: 20% to 25% height deformity
- Grade 2: 25% to 40% height deformity
- Grade 3: greater than 40% height deformity

A loss of more than 50% of the original height is indicative of instability[7] (Fig. 7.2).

On the AP view, the interpedicular distance, which is the distance measured between the pedicles, can be appreciated. The pedicles appear as ring-like structures on either side of the vertebral body. When compared with adjacent vertebrae, a widening of the space between each of the pedicles by more than 3 mm indicates a fracture of the vertebral body (Fig. 7.3). Oblique views can help determine alignment of the superior and inferior facets. The facet joints should be tightly apposed, symmetrical, and paired.

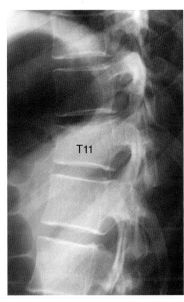

Fig. 7.2 Traumatic compression fracture of T11. This is a stable fracture because loss of anterior vertebral body height is not more than 50% when compared with the posterior vertebral height. (From Eiff MP, Hatch R, eds. Spine Fractures. In: *Fracture Management for Primary Care and Emergency Medicine.* 4th ed. Elsevier; 2019; Fig. 10.16.)

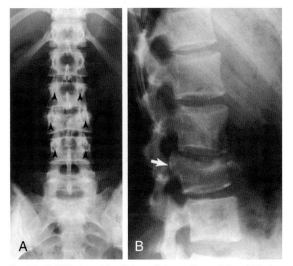

Fig. 7.3 (A) Widening of the distance between the pedicles of L3 when compared with the interpedicular distance of the adjacent vertebrae (*black arrowheads*). (B) Lateral view of the same patient showing a wedge fracture of L3 (*white arrow*). This is an unstable fracture because of the posterior displacement of bone fragments into the spinal canal. (From Nigel R, Berman L, Morley S, et al., eds. Thoracic & Lumbar Spine. In: *Accident and Emergency Radiology: A Survival Guide.* 3rd ed. Elsevier; 2014:377-402.)

The SJ system is indicated for use in the reduction of symptomatic OVCFs and traumatic vertebral compression fractures (type A fractures according to the AO/Magerl classification) with or without posterior instrumental fixation.[10]

CONTRAINDICATIONS

Absolute contraindications to vertebroplasty: asymptomatic vertebral compression fracture, active osteomyelitis of the target vertebra, coagulopathy that is not amenable to correction, allergy to cement used in procedure, and fractures that compromise the spinal canal.[11] Relative contraindications: significant central canal narrowing from retropulsion of bony fragment, epidural tumor, systemic infection, or interruption of the posterior cortex of the vertebral body.[11]

PERIOPERATIVE AND POSTOPERATIVE CONSIDERATIONS

Patients with OVCFs should be evaluated with a thorough history and physical exam, along with radiographic studies. It is important that the patient's symptoms are concordant with the level of fracture because compression fractures can be asymptomatic. A detailed neurological examination should be performed to diagnose any new or document underlying neurological compromise. Medication history should be reviewed, especially regarding opioid pain medications, anticoagulation, and anti-platelet medications.

In the postoperative period, patients are instructed to avoid strenuous activity, including bending, pushing, stretching, or pulling movements, for several weeks.

Procedural Steps

Patient evaluation should include the following preoperative steps.[12]

1. Assess the fracture, including fracture type.
2. Evaluate vertebral measurements: It is important to assess vertebral body length to determine the largest implant size that can be safely expanded in the vertebral body. Similarly, it is also critical to measure pedicle diameter (Fig. 7.4).
3. Gauge fracture mobility.
4. Target optimal implant placement: The SpineJack system is available in three implant kit

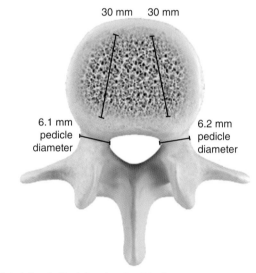

Fig.7.4 Vertebral body length and pedicle diameter measurements must be taken to determine implant size. (From Stryker Corporation. Spinejack System. https://strykerivs.com/products/families/spinejack-system.)

sizes: 4.2 mm, 5.0 mm, and 5.8 mm (Fig. 7.5). The various sizes accommodate for the various anatomy and fracture types. If the pedicle width measures between 5.0 and 5.8 mm, the recommended kit size is 4.2 mm; for pedicle diameters measuring between 5.8 and 6.6 mm,

a 5.0-mm kit size is recommended; for pedicle diameters of 6.6 or greater, the recommended kit size is 5.8 mm. It is preferred for the pedicle diameter to be 0.8 mm larger than the desired size of the implant in order to ensure safe placement of the implant (Fig. 7.6).

4.2 mm implant

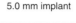

5.0 mm implant

5.8 mm implant

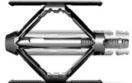
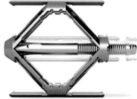

Control

The SpineJack system allows you to take full control of implant placement and expansion. Through bipedicular access and a series of cannulated steps, you achieve ideal positioning based on your assessment of the fracture type. The SpineJack implant expands in a craniocaudal direction, combatting the compression forces of the spine with up to 1,000 newtons of expansion force. It's power and precision, met with uncompromising control.

Restore

Restoring anatomy is paramount when it comes to fracture treatment, and the SpineJack system maximizes every millimeter. Osteoporotic VCF treatment outcomes are heavily tied to the amount of height restored and the SpineJack system now gives you the tools and the confidence to truly restore vertebral body height like never before.

Protect

Benefits of the SpineJack system are both immediate and lasting. The SpineJack system projects against adjacent level fractures, which may occur due to changes in the load distributed to adjacent vertebral bodies after an osteoporotic compression fracture. It's longterm protection that's been a long time coming.

Fig. 7.5 Implant sizes. (From Stryker Corporation. SpineJack System. https://strykerivs.com/products/families/spinejack-system.)

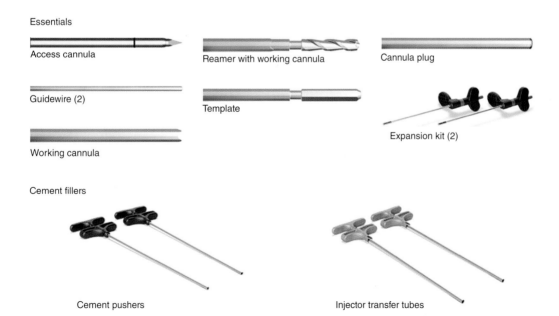

Fig. 7.6 Essential instruments and cement fillers. (From Stryker Corporation. SpineJack System. https://strykerivs.com/products/families/spinejack-system.)

INTRAOPERATIVE STEPS (FIG. 7.7)

1. Using a bilateral transpedicular approach, two 11-gauge cannulas are inserted and advanced to the posterior one-third of the vertebral body.
2. The guidewire is inserted into each cannula and advanced to the midpoint of the vertebral body; subsequently, the access cannulas are removed.
3. Using the pathway of the guidewire, the reamers are inserted and advanced until they are seated entirely within the vertebral body.
4. The templates are then introduced to clean the implant site and to confirm the length of the implant.
5. Two SJs are inserted into the vertebral body (unexpanded).
6. The SJs are then expanded to reduce the fracture and thereby restore the anatomy and vertebral body height. The implants expand in a craniocaudal fashion, combatting the compression forces of the spine with up to 1000 newtons of expansion force.
7. Next, the SJs are expanded and cement is injected to stabilize the fracture.

Complications

Postoperative follow-up is necessary to monitor for potential complications. Although rare, complications related to SJ implantation may include infection, hematoma, paralysis, persistent or worsening pain, pulmonary embolism, accidental cement extravasation, or allergic reaction to bone cement (PMMA) or contrast.[13-15] Late complications can also include subsequent vertebral compression fractures in adjacent levels.[13]

Cement leakage from the vertebral body is the most common complication, with an incidence of 8.1%, but is rarely symptomatic (0.09% symptomatic rate).[16] Paralysis is a serious but rare complication (0.16%) that can occur with this procedure if the spinal cord is injured, such as with malpositioning of the instrument or with cement extravasation into the spinal canal.[14,15] Furthermore, if cement accidentally leaks into the spinal canal or to nearby nerve roots it can also result in spinal stenosis and persistent or worsening pain as well as numbness, tingling, or weakness.[13-15] A pulmonary embolism can potentially occur if cement happens to enter a vertebral vein and travel into the lung resulting in obstruction, which occurred in 0.17% of all clinical scenarios.[13,16] The overall mortality associated with this procedure is 4.4%, with perioperative mortality being 0.13%.[16]

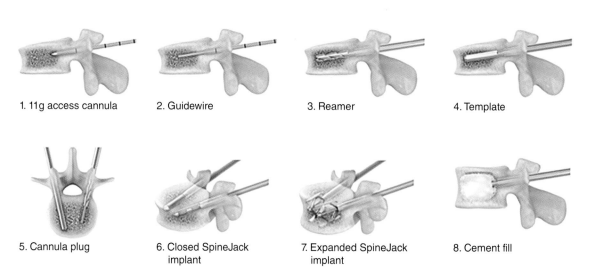

1. 11g access cannula   2. Guidewire   3. Reamer   4. Template

5. Cannula plug   6. Closed SpineJack implant   7. Expanded SpineJack implant   8. Cement fill

Fig. 7.7 Illustration of steps for SpineJack procedure. (Courtesy Stryker Corporation.)

REFERENCES

1. Alexandru D, So W. Evaluation and management of vertebral compression fractures. *Perm J*. 2012;16(4):46-51.
2. Wood KB, Li W, Lebl DR, et al. Management of thoracolumbar spine fractures. *Spine J*. 2014;14(1):145-164.
3. Manson NA, Phillips FM. Minimally invasive techniques for the treatment of osteoporotic vertebral fractures. *Instr Course Lect*. 2007;56:273-285.
4. Krüger A, Oberkircher L, Figiel J, et al. Height restoration of osteoporotic vertebral compression fractures using different intravertebral reduction devices: a cadaveric study. *Spine J*. 2015;15(5):1092-1098.
5. Krüger A, Baroud A, Noriega D, et al. Height restoration and maintenance after treating unstable osteoporotic vertebral compression fractures by cement augmentation is dependent on the cement volume used. *Clin Biomech (Bristol, Avon)*. 2013;28(7): 725-730.
6. Noriega D, Marcia S, Theumann N, et al. A prospective, international, randomized, noninferiority study comparing an implantable titanium vertebral augmentation device versus balloon kyphoplasty in the reduction of vertebral compression fractures (SAKOS study). *Spine J*. 2019;19(11):1782-1795.
7. Eiff MP, Hatch R. *Fracture Management for Primary Care and Emergency Medicine*. 4th ed. Elsevier; 2019.
8. Raby N, Berman L, Morley S, et al. *Accident and Emergency Radiology: A Survival Guide*. Elsevier; 2014.
9. Genant HK, Wu CY, van Kuijk C, et al. Vertebral fracture assessment using a semiquantitative technique. *J Bone Miner Res*. 1993;8(9):1137-1148.
10. Guglielmi G, Andreula C, Muto M, Gilula LA. Percutaneous vertebroplasty: indications, contraindications, technique, and complications. *Acta Radiol*. 2005;46(3):256-268.
11. Appel NB, Gilula LA. Percutaneous vertebroplasty in patients with spinal canal compromise. *AJR Am J Roentgenol*. 2004;182(4): 947-951.
12. Stryker. *SpineJack System*. https://strykerivs.com/products/families/spinejack-system. Accessed October 27, 2021.
13. Noriega D, Maestretti G, Renaud C, et al. Clinical performance and safety of 108 SpineJack implantations: 1-year results of a prospective multicentre single-arm registry study. *Biomed Res Int*. 2015;2015:173872.
14. Robinson Y, Tschöke SK, Stahel PF, et al. Complications and safety aspects of kyphoplasty for osteoporotic vertebral fractures: a prospective follow-up study in 102 consecutive patients. *Patient Saf Surg*. 2008;2:2.
15. Taylor RS, Fritzell P, Taylor RJ. Balloon kyphoplasty in the management of vertebral compression fractures: an updated systematic review and meta-analysis. *Eur Spine J*. 2007;16: 1085-1100.
16. Choe DH, Marom EM, Ahrar K, Truong MT, Madewell JE. Pulmonary embolism of polymethyl methacrylate during percutaneous vertebroplasty and kyphoplasty. *Am J Roentgenol*. 2004;183:1097-1102.

Chapter 8

Radiofrequency Ablation for Metastatic Bone Lesions With Vertebral Augmentation

Gabrielle Frisenda, Tariq Malik, and Ahmed Malik

Introduction

Bone is the third most common site of tumor metastasis after lung and liver. Of all bones, the spine is the most frequent site of metastasis (Table 8.1). Osseous metastatic lesions can be seen in up to 80% of cancer patients at the time of their death, with up to half of these metastases located in the spine.[1] This is thought to be related to the vascularity and hematopoietic role of the vertebrae. The cancer causes pain and erosion of the bone, leading to fracture (Table 8.2). The pain from these metastases can be debilitating for patients, impairing patient mobility and leading to depression and a decrease in quality of life.[2] These lesions are traditionally managed with a combination of radiation therapy (mainstay), chemotherapy, medical therapy with bisphosphonates or targeted bone agents,[3] and occasionally surgical intervention should the patient be a candidate.

These interventions do have their limitations, however. Incomplete or lack of pain relief in patients receiving radiotherapy for painful bone metastasis has been documented in a large meta-analysis study in 60% and 23% of patients respectively.[4] Pain relief may also take as long as 4 to 6 weeks to be fully effective.[5] Complications from these treatments are not to be ignored as patients undergoing radiotherapy have documented fracture rates as high as 39%.[6] In patients with longer life expectancy, recurrence of symptoms after initial response has been observed as well.[7] Additional radiotherapy is often avoided in these patients due to risk of radiation myelopathy. These limitations have allowed radiofrequency ablation (RFA) with vertebral augmentation to demonstrate its ability to provide accelerated pain control faster with fewer complications when compared with the current standard of care.

Multiple studies have demonstrated the role of RFA of metastatic bone lesions followed by vertebral augmentation in reducing pain scores. The benefits include improvement in mood, improved quality of life, and a reduction in opioid use.[8] Safety and efficacy of RFA of metastatic bone lesions has also been demonstrated. One study examined 87 patients experiencing pain from metastatic disease in the spine and/or sacrum who underwent RFA with subsequent cementoplasty. The outcome was a rapid and statistically significant improvement in pain within 3 days of the procedure with sustained relief at 6 months in the majority of patients.[9]

TABLE 8.1 Tumors That Metastasize to the Spine
Prostate
Breast
Lung
Thyroid
Renal
Colorectal
Myeloma
Melanoma

TABLE 8.2 Type of Lesion	
Osteolytic	70%
Osteoblastic	8%
Mixed	21%

The analgesic effect of RFA is attributed to destruction of tumor cells and nociceptive nerves, lower tumor-mediated cytokine release, and delays in tumor progression to the periosteum.[10] Subsequent cementoplasty allows for stabilization of fractured trabeculae and may prevent vertebral body collapse as a result of ablation or tumor invasion.[11] Patient selection, workup, contraindications, and the procedure itself are described in the following sections.

Background

The biological effect of radiofrequency (RF) waves on tissue was described by the French physiologist Jaques D'Arsonval (1851–1940) in the late 19th century (1891). However, use of RF energy in medicine came with the invention of the Bovie knife. Rossi et al.[12] independently described using RF thermal therapy to treat a tumor nodule in the liver in 1992. Since then, this mode of therapy has grown in popularity and has been used for tumor ablation worldwide.

PHYSICS OF RADIOFREQUENCY

RF waves are part of the electromagnetic spectrum. Electromagnetic waves are massless vibrating photons that carry varying amounts of energy depending on their frequency. Waves with frequency ranges of 30 Hz to 300 GHz are called *radio waves*. RF ablative devices work in the 450- to 500-kHz range. RFA causes coagulative necrosis by inducing thermal heating of tissue. An RF machine emits RF waves through an electrode, the probe in this case. The alternating current fed to the generator causes the generator to create a high-frequency alternating electromagnetic field. The dipoles in the electromagnetic field are forced to align within the field. This alternating field causes the adjacent dipoles—in this case, the water molecules surrounding the tissues—to vibrate at the frequency of the RF waves, resulting in agitation. This agitation generates heat within the tissue. The heat generated by the friction, when high enough, leads to protein denaturation and cell death. The electrode itself never gets hot; all of the heat is generated within the tissue. The tissue biopsy examined under the microscope will reveal coagulative necrosis. The size of the thermal burn depends on tissue ability to handle the heat and the power of the device to deliver it. In general, the

TABLE 8.3 Temperature and Time to Cell Death

Temperature (Celsius)	Time to Cell Death
< 45	No cell death, hyperemia
46	60 minutes
50–52	6 minutes
60–100	A few seconds
> 105	Vaporization, carbonization

size is proportional to the net energy deposited. Temperature above 45° C is lethal to mammalian cells in 15 minutes or more. At temperatures above 50° C, this time is reduced to a few minutes. At temperatures above 100° C, tissue vaporizes instantly, creating air bubbles, which then restrict the conduction of heat and, thus, limit burn size (Table 8.3). Therefore slow delivery of heat at 50° C to 90° C to the surrounding tissue creates optimal size burn.

TYPE OF RADIOFREQUENCY ABLATION

RF energy can be delivered either via unipolar electrode or bipolar electrode. In a unipolar electrode, the electromagnetic field is created between the electrode (cathode) and the grounding pad (the returning electrode or anode). This setup produces intense heat generation at the electrode tip, causing localized charring, as seen in a surgical Bovie knife. Unipolar RF does not deposit energy uniformly within the tissue, and the uneven heat deposition gets worse when the electrode diameter is increased. Hence, unipolar electrodes are not suitable for ablation of large lesions. In bipolar RF, both electrodes are present on the same needle or catheter and the electromagnetic field is created between the two electrodes. This yields a more controlled dispersion of heat and a more predictable lesion.

Bipolar RF device development has led to the safe application of this therapy to tumor lesions within the spine while avoiding any nerve or spinal cord damage.

TYPES OF ELECTRODES
Cooled Versus Non-cooled Probes

Goldberg et al. first reported use of chilled saline during RF, which reduced charring and impedance, resulting in increased tumor volume ablation.[13] The cooled RF device is commercially available and is manufactured by Medtronic (OsteoCool™). Using ice water (0° C), the electrode tip temperature stays around 15° C, and charring can be prevented altogether. If room temperature water is used, the tip of the probe cools down to 35° C, which prevents charring if the generator power is kept at 50 W or less. If the electrode tip is cooled to 45° C, all benefits of cooling (increased lesion size and absence of charring) are lost.

Navigational Bipolar Probe

The SpineSTAR Ablation system—its RF electrode has an active navigational tip that can be maneuvered into difficult spots, such as the posterior part of the vertebral body.

Perfused Bipolar Electrode

A saline- or dextrose-based solution is injected into tissue through the electrode during RFA. Saline works by improving heat conductivity as well as increasing ion availability within the tissue to generate more heat. Hypertonic saline increases the lesion size much more than normal saline.[14]

Patient Selection/Workup

RFA is approved by the US Food and Drug Administration for patients suffering from pain due to malignancy in the bone. The National Comprehensive Cancer Network (NCCN) endorses RFA as a method for improving malignant bony pain.[15]

A patient is a candidate for this therapy if suffering from localized back pain due to malignancy. It can be locally curative if the ablation takes out the lesion completely, preventing local recurrence. It is also useful in preventing impending fracture or collapse of a vertebral body when ablation is followed by cementoplasty.

Patient evaluation includes complete history and physical examination, with focus on determining the pathology of the lesion and whether the tumor is chemo- or radiosensitive so that the best combination therapy can be planned. Look for any sign of nerve or cord compression. Stability of the spine or possibility of cord compression should elicit surgical consultation (Table 8.4).

Imaging is imperative. Magnetic resonance imaging (MRI) with contrast is done to evaluate the size and location of the lesion in order to plan placement of the

TABLE 8.4 Elements of Evaluation

Patient Evaluation
- Pain
  - Intensity
  - Medication
  - Coexisting medical issues
  - Life expectancy
  - Comorbidities
  - Performance status
- Spine
  - Fracture
  - Cord compression
  - Epidural extension
  - Spine instability

Treatment Options
- Chemotherapy or radiotherapy
- Prior surgery or procedures at the level
- Surgery
- Clinical trial or not

RF catheter. Look for any expansion of the lesion into the surrounding tissue, especially the epidural space and the pedicles, as this can increase the probability of nerve damage from the heat during RFA. If there is a contraindication to MRI, nuclear scintigraphic bone scan with single-photon emission computed tomography (SPECT) is the next best option. CT of the spine is useful in evaluating the integrity of the vertebrae.

It is important to screen for coagulopathy, systemic infection, and relevant metabolic abnormalities. Additional tests should be ordered when clinically warranted. All anticoagulant therapies should be held, as the procedure is considered high risk for bleeding.

INDICATIONS

RFA is considered under the following circumstances:

1. Poorly controlled lesion-related pain that is nonresponsive to opioid therapy.
2. The tumor is radioresistant and expanding.
3. The tumor is radiosensitive but dose limits have been reached.
4. The tumor is radiosensitive but pain is debilitating and urgent intervention is needed.
5. When chemotherapy cannot be interrupted even to have radiation therapy or surgery.
6. Patients in whom invasive surgical procedures are not warranted given short life expectancy and/or comorbidities.

7. There is a risk of myelosuppression from radiation or chemotherapy.
8. As a part of combination therapy (surgery + RF or radiation + RF, or chemo + RF).

CONTRAINDICATIONS

- Patient refusal.
- Metastases associated with pathologic compression fracture with spinal instability.
- Metastases causing spinal cord compression.
- Highly vascular tumors (renal tumor, melanoma).
- Sclerotic lesions (prostate tumor, postradiation sclerosis).
- Patient-reported or documented history of allergy to bone cement.
- Bleeding disorder or current/recent use of anticoagulation that cannot be corrected.
- Any metal in the bone that can result in heat damage.
- Medically unstable, active spinal infection.

CONSENT

Informed consent is obtained. The benefits of procedure are effective and prompt pain control, spine stability, and potential to locally cure the tumor.

The risks come from the needle, RF therapy, and from cement injection. The risks from the needle and cement are covered separately in this book. There is a risk of unintended heat damage from RFA to the surrounding tissue, especially nerve roots and the spinal cord, which is irreversible. The risk is very low but real. Various strategies have been used to eliminate this risk, which will be discussed later. The tumor may recur after the ablation therapy.

Procedural Technique

SETUP

The procedure is done in a sterile fashion. It can be done with light sedation; however, depending on patient health and extent of discomfort from positioning, deeper sedation or general anesthesia may be needed.

POSITION

The patient is placed prone on the operating room table. If the patient is unable to tolerate prone positioning, oblique prone positioning can be considered. It is important to ensure that the intended vertebral level is clearly visible with fluoroscopic imaging. It is especially a concern in the thoracic area, where the patient's arm can obscure the lateral view. If possible, the arm should be positioned above the head.

ANTISEPTIC PRECAUTIONS

Antibiotic prophylaxis should be administered to patients using either cefazolin 1 to 2 g or clindamycin 600 mg if the patient has a penicillin allergy. The skin is cleaned with a sterile antiseptic solution. Most commonly, a combination of 2% chlorhexidine gluconate in 70% isopropyl alcohol is used, which is effective for both rapid and persistent reduction of bacterial load for a broad spectrum of organisms. Prep the skin and drape the back widely. The washed skin is covered with an antimicrobial surgical-incise-adhesive drape. The drapes have antimicrobial activity. It slowly releases iodophor onto the skin in order to provide continuous, broad-spectrum antimicrobial activity throughout the surgical procedure.

PROCEDURE STEPS

1. Position fluoroscopy C-arms in both anteroposterior (AP) and lateral positions. Identify the appropriate vertebral levels. Optimize the AP and lateral views of the vertebra. In the AP view, the pedicles should be clearly visualized and the end plates should be aligned with the spinous process equidistant from each pedicle. In the lateral view (Fig. 8.1), the two pedicles should

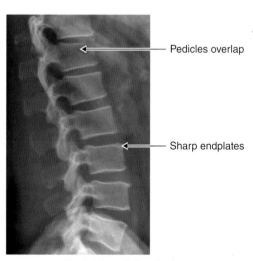

Pedicles overlap

Sharp endplates

Fig. 8.1 Lateral view of spine.

be superimposed, the end plates should appear as one line, and the posterior vertebral body wall should be crisp.

2. RFA is performed in conjunction with cementoplasty. The three main components of the procedure are as follows.
   a. Accessing the vertebral body with one or two trocars/cannula (10–13 F)
   b. Placing one or two RFA probes via the cannula.
   c. Cement injection with or without kyphoplasty.

3. The components (a) and (b) part of the procedure have been covered in Chapter 4 and will be reviewed only briefly here.

4. Selecting the skin entry point is extremely important. The two overarching principles in planning the cannula trajectory are as follows.
   a. Safely enter the vertebral body via the pedicle without violating the spinal canal.
   b. The trajectory of the cannula should optimize placement of the RF probe to maximize size of the lesion.

5. Two RFA systems are commercially available, OsteoCool (Medtronic, Minneapolis, MN) and SpineSTAR (Merit Medical, South Jordan, UT). The RF probe placement is different for each system.

OsteoCool

1. After confirmation of the appropriate level, create a small skin incision using a #15 blade.

2. Insert the bone trocar(s) using a mallet. Advance into the portion of the vertebral body necessary for access to the lesion with a transpedicular or parapedicular approach and guidance with fluoroscopy. A transpedicular trajectory passes through the entire length of the pedicle into the vertebral body. This approach shields adjacent neural and vascular structures but can limit the ability to achieve a midline needle tip position. Figs. 8.2 and 8.3 demonstrate the transpedicular approach.

In the parapedicular trajectory, the lateral wall of the pedicle is penetrated, which often

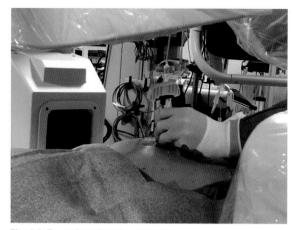

Fig. 8.2 Trocar insertion via transpedicular approach on patient in prone position.

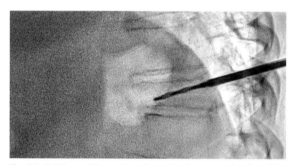

Fig. 8.3 Drill is used to create a channel and measure the size of the radiofrequency probe.

makes midline needle tip positioning easier to attain.

Once the trocar is positioned in the vertebral body, a bone biopsy can be done if needed for diagnostic purposes.

3. A drill from the commercial kit is used to create a channel for the RF probe and to gauge the size of the RF probe for ablation. The procedure is repeated on the other side. The markings on the drill are color coded to help decide which size RF probe will be needed for ablation (see Fig. 8.3)

4. The RF probe comes in four sizes. The size refers to the active part of the probe tip.
   a. 7 mm (yellow)
   b. 10 mm (blue)
   c. 15 mm (orange)
   d. 20 mm (green)

   The larger the probe size, bigger the lesion (Fig. 8.4).

5. Once the probes are placed through the cannula on each side, their proper position can be confirmed with imaging. The latching mechanism (Fig. 8.5) ensures that the probes are well within the body and that the active tip of the probe is not touching the cannula or too close to the posterior vertebral wall.

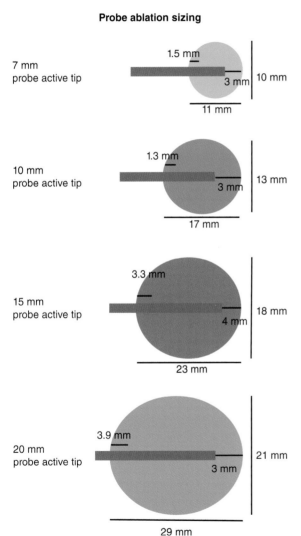

Probe ablation sizing

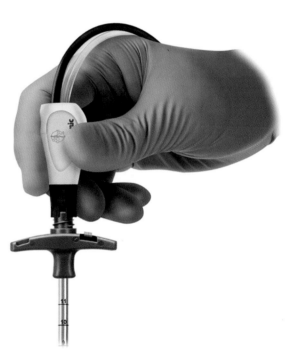

Fig. 8.5 Medtronic latching mechanism; probe located within the trocar. (From Medtronic. OsteoCool Radiofrequency Ablation System. https://www.medtronic.com/us-en/healthcare-professionals/products/spinal-orthopaedic/tumor-management/osteocool-ablation-system-rf.html.)

Fig. 8.4 Ablation probe sizing per OsteoCool Radiofrequency Ablation System. (From Medtronic. OsteoCool Radiofrequency Ablation System. https://www.medtronic.com/us-en/healthcare-professionals/products/spinal-orthopaedic/tumor-management/osteocool-ablation-system-rf.html.)

The probe is connected to the water pump and generator. RFA is completed with the Medtronic protocol (Fig. 8.6). The machine displays the temperature (in Celsius), power (watts) being generated, and the resistance (ohms). The time cycle is different for each probe size.

a. 7-mm probe (6:30-minute ablation cycle)
b. 10-mm probe (7:30-minute ablation cycle)
c. 15-mm probe (11:30-minute ablation cycle)
d. 20-mm probe (15:00-minute ablation cycle)

The OsteoCool generator has a built-in bone algorithm that utilizes time, ramp rate, power and

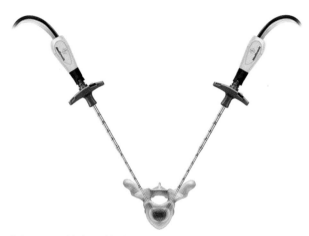

Fig. 8.6 Medtronic animation of radiofrequency ablation with dual probe via transpedicular approach. (From Medtronic. OsteoCool Radiofrequency Ablation System. https://www.medtronic.com/us-en/healthcare-professionals/products/spinal-orthopaedic/tumor-management/osteocool-ablation-system-rf.html.)

temperature (Fig. 8.7) to achieve a standard ablation zone (Fig. 8.8). The zone can be customized by adjusting these four variables. The customized ablation zones are used in the pelvis, sacrum, and ribs. A standard ablation zone is appropriate for vertebral body ablations.

6. After completion of RFA, insert the kyphoplasty balloon via each cannula within the vertebral body under fluoroscopic guidance. Position the cannula and balloon within the vertebral body. The radio marker on the balloon helps to ensure that it is well within the vertebral body (Fig. 8.9).

7. Inflate the balloon with radiopaque dye in increments of 0.25 to 0.5 mL (Fig. 8.10). Pay close attention to the balloon pressure so that it

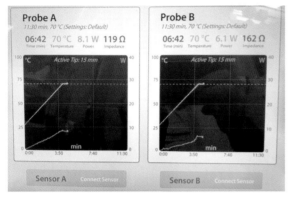

Fig. 8.7 OsteoCool radiofrequency generator interface with settings (time, ramp rate, power [watts], and temperature).

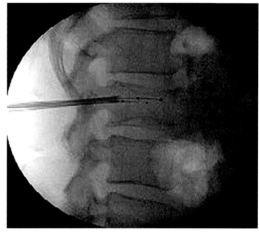

Fig. 8.9 Fluoroscopic view of the spine with balloon radio-markers within the vertebral body.

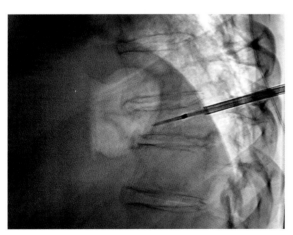

Fig. 8.8 Lateral view of spine, radiofrequency ablation probe and ablation zone.

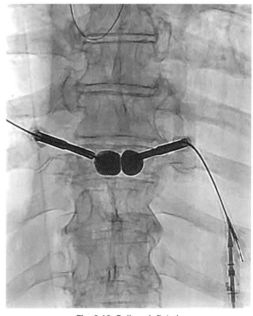

Fig. 8.10 Balloon inflated.

does not exceed approved PSI limits (400 mm Hg). If there is a compression fracture and height restoration is intended, then keep inflating until limits of expansion or other end points are reached. In the absence of compression fracture, this step can be skipped by going directly to cementoplasty.

Balloon inflation is stopped when the upper limit of volume or pressure is reached or height restoration is achieved.

8. Leave the balloon inflated for approximately 3 minutes while the high-viscosity radiopaque bone cement is prepared. Once prepared, deflate and remove the balloon.

9. Inject the methyl methacrylate cement on both sides via the introducer under continuous fluoroscopic guidance. Ensure that there is no cement extravasation into the epidural space or outside of the vertebral body.

10. Once the bone cement is hardened, slowly remove the cannulas under fluoroscopic guidance to ensure no unneeded extravasation.

11. Close the incisions with Dermabond or 4-0 synthetic absorbable sutures. Apply adhesive strips and cover the skin incision with water resistant dressing for 24 to 48 hours.

Optimal Probe Position

Ablation therapy effectiveness relies on the total destruction of the lesion. This requires ensuring that the lesion and a margin of healthy tissue are with the thermal ablation zone. Optimal probe positioning requires that the largest possible probe be used, the two probes are positioned at the distance that produces the largest lesion, and the probes are positioned in the part of the vertebral body that has the tumor (see Fig. 8.1). Thus, meticulous mapping out the tumor using MRI is crucial for correct probe placement within the tumor.

If the tumor is large, the probes can be repositioned to place another burn to extend the lesion. OsteoCool probes are not conducive to accessing the lesion in the posterior part of the vertebral body. Creation of the lesion within 1 cm of the posterior wall or with the pedicle should be avoided without extra safeguards to prevent thermal spinal cord injury. This will be discussed later in the chapter.

OSTEOCOOL SYSTEM

The OsteoCool system generates an ablative lesion by generating heat in the tissue. The machine senses impedance from the tip of the probe and adjusts the power to maintain a constant current flow to generate heat. The expected lesion size (Fig. 8.11) is based on mathematical and experimental models in which heat is slowly ramped up and then maintained for a specified number of minutes. The lesion size is based on the edges of the tissue where temperature will reach 50° C. There is no real time temperature monitoring of surrounding tissue.

The OsteoCool system has the capability to connect to a thermocouple, a temperature sensor that can be used to prevent damage to the nearby vital structures.

SpineSTAR™ TUMOR ABLATION SYSTEM

The SpineSTAR system has a bipolar RF probe with a navigation ablation instrument. It is a unipedicular system; RFA is performed by accessing only one pedicle. The overall procedure steps are very similar to the OsteoCool system by Medtronic.

1. After prepping and draping the patient, the correct vertebral level is visualized in the AP and lateral fluoroscopic views.

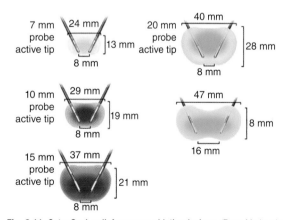

Fig. 8.11 OsteoCool radiofrequency ablation lesions. (From Medtronic. OsteoCool Radiofrequency Ablation System. https://www.medtronic.com/us-en/healthcare-professionals/products/spinal-orthopaedic/tumor-management/osteocool-ablation-system-rf.html.)

2. Local anesthetic is used to numb the skin—including the deeper tissues all the way to the periosteum.

3. An introducer from the commercial kit is placed within the vertebral body through the pedicle using the same principles and precautions as previously mentioned.

4. Once in place, the SpineSTAR ablation instrument is placed into the tumor of the vertebral body. The active tip is extended into the lesion. The ablation instrument can be steered in any direction by turning the knob at the handle of the device along with rotating the ablation instrument (Fig. 8.12).

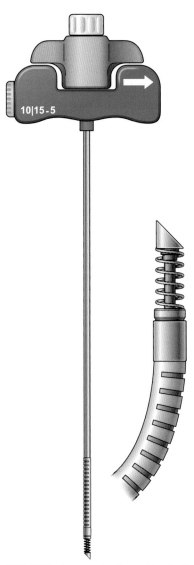

Fig. 8.12 SpineSTAR ablation instrument with overlying flexible steerable tip.

5. Once the device is appropriately positioned, the electrode tip is extended out by turning the knob at the handle and is connected to the generator to produce the thermal ablative burn (Fig. 8.13).

6. The ablation instrument has two thermocouples. The generator is set to turn off when the temperature at the proximal sensor reaches 50° C. The probe has navigational capability; it can be withdrawn and repositioned in a different area of the tumor to produce multiple overlapping lesions to ensure a complete ablation of the tumor. In one study, 4.3 lesions were made per vertebral level, on average.[1]

7. The working ablation cannula comes in two sizes (Fig. 8.14).
   a. SpineSTAR 5 | 10
      - Distal thermocouple at 5 mm
      - Proximal thermocouple at 10 mm
      - Maximum ablation zone ~2 × 1.5 cm

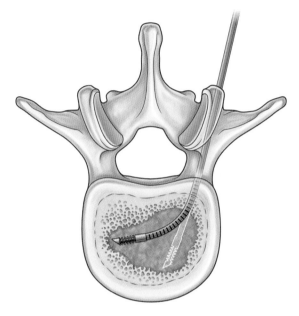

Fig. 8.13 Radiofrequency ablation zone with extension of electrode tip.

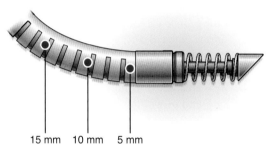

15 mm   10 mm   5 mm

Fig. 8.14 SpineSTAR configurations.

TABLE 8.5 Catheter Type and Associated Ablation Region Sizes

RF Catheter Type	Ablation Size When Temperature Reaches 50° C
SpineSTAR 5/10	Distal TC (5 mm) ≈ 1 × 0.75 cm Proximal TC (10 mm) ≈ 2 × 1.5 cm
SpineSTAR 10/15	Distal TC (10 mm) ≈ 2 × 1.5 cm Proximal TC (15 mm) ≈ 3 × 2 cm

TC, Thermocouple.

   b. SpineSTAR 10 | 15
- Distal thermocouple at 10 mm
- Proximal thermocouple at 15 mm
- Maximum ablation zone ~3 × 2 cm

8. Depending on the size of the ablation instrument, ablation size can be controlled and is useful in ablating lesions in small places such as the pedicle without causing unwanted nerve damage (Table 8.5)
9. Optimal position of the probe depends on tumor location within the vertebral body.
10. Once ablation is complete, cementoplasty is done with or without kyphoplasty.

Unique Features of the STAR Navigational System

The STAR tumor ablation system has three unique features that differentiate it from the OsteoCool system.

1. The system is designed to ablate tumor with one probe instead of placing two probes in the vertebral body via each pedicle. The navigational capability of the probe allows the operator to steer the probe into any part of the body. Even a large lesion can be ablated by repositioning the probe into a different part of the lesion sequentially and repeating the burn cycle.
2. The probe has two temperature sensors, distal and proximal. The machine is designed to keep heating up the tissue until the proximal sensor (the one farthest from the tip) senses 50° C. The sensor represents the outer edge of the ablation zone. There is no set time limit; whenever the temperature is achieved, the ablation cycle is complete (Fig. 8.15).

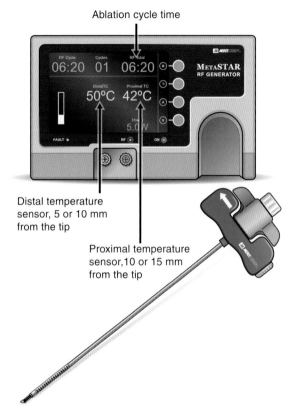

Fig. 8.15 Merit generator and the ablation instrument with navigational tip.

Labels: Ablation cycle time — Distal temperature sensor, 5 or 10 mm from the tip — Proximal temperature sensor, 10 or 15 mm from the tip

3. The system is designed to ablate lesions in the posterior part of the vertebral body. This is possible due to the navigational capability of the bipolar probe and the thermocouple sensors on the probe. The probe is placed at least 1 cm from the posterior wall to avoid thermal injury to the spinal cord.

Strategies to Minimize Risk of Spinal Cord Damage During Radiofrequency Ablation

Spinal cord or nerve root damage is the most concerning side effect or complication of RF therapy to treat tumor within the vertebral body. Neurodeficit is immediately seen at the end of the therapy and is usually permanent. A temperature at or above 50° C is lethal within minutes. Transfer of heat to the spinal cord is the most common cause of this complication, which is a result of placement of the bipolar RF probe too close to the posterior wall. Erosion or cracks in the posterior vertebral body wall facilitates heat transfer, resulting in high heat transfer to the spinal cord. Three interventions are described in literature for neuroprotection when RF therapy is applied in the pedicle or close to the posterior vertebral wall.

1. Intraprocedure neuroelectrical monitoring: The evoked motor and sensory evoked potentials detect damage when these parameters change (increase in evoked motor potential threshold by 100 V), lower amplitude of compound sensory evoked potential form baseline, and/or increase in latency of nerves (increase in latency by 10% or drop in mAmp by 60%). These parameters are very sensitive and specific.[16]
2. CO_2 insufflation: CO_2 is an inert gas with insulating properties, used for hydro section. A needle is placed between the tissue to be saved and the burn lesion that will be created. Commercial kits are available.[17]
3. Cold sterile water/D_5 irrigation: Just like CO_2, cold irrigation done by placing an epidural or spinal needle through the foramen in the anterior epidural space prevents high heat transfer to the spinal cord.[18]

Complications

As thermal RFA continues to emerge as a legitimate alternative to the current standard of care, it is important to review the adverse events that have been associated with this technology. Of the documented complications, thermal injury of neural structures carries with it a significant degree of morbidity and may result in weakness, paralysis, paresthesias, dysesthesia, or anesthesia of all sensations. While frequently temporary, these injuries may be permanent.

Huntoon et al.[19] identified 17 studies that included 399 cases of RF thermal ablation and found that the majority supported the safety and efficacy of RFA. Findings included no major neurological events and significant improvement in pain, especially in patients with unresectable spine tumors refractory to radiotherapy and chemotherapy. Of the 399 cases, only 19 cases

reported possible neurological complications from the RFA procedure. Radicular pain most commonly caused by cement leakage accounted for the majority of these complications. Transient symptoms related to bowel and bladder incontinence, worsening of preexisting extremity weakness, and new onset of leg weakness that partially improved with conservative management made up the rest. In this same paper, Huntoon et al. also described the first and only documented case of permanent paralysis in a patient who underwent RFA for metastatic spine lesions. The paralysis was thought to be due to thermal damage of the ventral nerve roots after inaccurate placement of the RFA probe or more extensive zones of thermal ablation than anticipated.

As more data emerges, it is crucial to be aware of the complications and be ready to respond to them. A full neurological assessment following the procedure is important to rule out serious adverse outcomes. Should new-onset weakness or changes in sensation or bowel or bladder function be noted, consider immediate CT to look for any evidence of new fractures or cement extravasation into the spinal canal or spinal foramina. MRI would also be useful to assess for any signs of focal stenosis or spinal cord compression or infarct. Gadolinium-enhanced T1-weighted MRI specifically looking for any enhancement of the nerves suggestive of thermal injury can also be done if the prior imaging modalities cannot account for the changes on physical exam. Electromyography can also be helpful in eliciting causes.

Other complications to be aware of are the following:

- Delayed pain relief (4–6 weeks) or no pain relief
- Patients with longer life expectancy may experience recurrent symptoms after initial response
- Fracture of ablated vertebrae that were not augmented
- Pulmonary embolism from cement leak
- Allergic reaction, hypotension, depressed cardiac function due to cement injection
- Pneumothorax
- Bleeding (e.g., paraspinal hematoma)

Discussion

As the population ages, the incidence of cancer increases. Therapeutic options are improving and patients are surviving longer. This is bound to increase prevalence of advanced metastatic cancer and, invariably, cancerous bone lesions. Currently, radiotherapy are chemotherapy are first-line treatments for bone pain. Both have their limitations. Even in optimal situations, the analgesic effects of these therapies are not seen for days to weeks, may delay other interventions, or may cause some other untoward side effect. RF therapy has a proven safety and effectiveness record worldwide. Numerous soft tissue and bony lesions have been successfully treated with it. RF therapy works by energizing the water within the tissue, which then heats up the tissue. RF therapy is locally curative by taking out the whole lesion. This is achieved by ablating 0.5 to 1 cm of surrounding healthy tissue, which may contain tumor cells, along with the tumor. Temperature above 45° C is lethal after several minutes; at 50° C or above, cell death occurs in a few minutes. The two commercially available devices based their predicted lesion size on achieving 50° C at the margin of the burn. The OsteoCool system achieves this by maintaining 70° C at the tip of bipolar electrode and sustaining that temperature long enough to allow heat to be deposited in the surrounding tissue at a far enough distance to achieve a predicted burn size, resulting in total ablation of the cancerous lesion. The water circulating through the RF probe keeps the temperature low to prevent buildup of an overly high temperature, preventing charring of the surrounding tissue. There is no real time measurement of temperature of the surrounding tissue nor is there a way to confirm whether the predicted size lesion has been produced. This can lead to nerve damage, thus, necessitates extra vigilance. The SpineSTAR system has a bipolar RF catheter. Its RFA protocol relies on sensing temperature at 10 or 15 mm from the active tip to determine the extent of the letter. This navigational aspect and the temperature sensing capability of the RF catheter make it the more versatile system.

RFA provides prompt, durable pain relief, along with curing the disease locally.[20] When combined with cementoplasty, RFA can prevent or treat fracture from the disease by strengthening the vertebral body. Its safety has been established in many trials.[6] When performed in conjunction with cementoplasty, it minimizes or eliminates spilling of tumor cells from kyphoplasty. It provides pain relief when radiation and chemotherapy have failed[21] and has a synergistic effect when combined with radiation therapy.[22] In general, stereotactic body radiotherapy (SBRT) is done before RFA with augmentation. SBRT has a curative effect, limiting or preventing tumor seeding from the RFA. If done after RFA, there is risk of seeding, which potentially limits the effectiveness of SBRT by distorting the target area.

Level of Evidence

RF therapy has not been evaluated in a double-blind, randomized fashion. All studies are either observational or prospective cohort studies. Based on these studies, there is level II evidence for RFA therapy for spine tumor in providing effective and durable analgesia.

Conclusion

RFA is a safe and effective technique. It should be done in conjunction with cementoplasty to prevent a fracture in the near future, especially if the spine has been treated with SBRT, which increases the risk of vertebral body fracture. It is locally curative when done properly, preventing recurrence of tumor at the site. It can provide pain relief when radiotherapy and chemotherapy have failed. It can greatly improve quality of life in cancer patients.

Billing

ICD DIAGNOSTIC CODES

D16.6	Benign neoplasm of vertebral column
D89.3	Neoplasm-related pain (acute, chronic)
C79.51 with pain code C89.3	Painful metastatic bone lesion

ICD-10-CM PROCEDURE CODES FOR HOSPITALS FOR INPATIENT PROCEDURES

0P543ZZ	Destruction of thoracic vertebra, percutaneous approach
0Q503ZZ	Destruction of lumbar vertebra, percutaneous approach

PHYSICIAN CODING

CPT codes for Ablation-A single CPT code identifies RFA of bone tumor, regardless of the site.

20982   Ablation therapy for reduction or eradication of one or more bone tumors (e.g., metastasis), including adjacent soft tissue when involved by tumor extension, percutaneous, including imaging guidance when performed; radiofrequency

REFERENCES

1. Anchala PR, Irving WD, Hillen TJ, et al. Treatment of metastatic spinal lesions with a navigational bipolar radiofrequency ablation device: a multicenter retrospective study. *Pain Physician.* 2014;17(4):317-327.
2. Roque IFM, Martinez-Zapata MJ, Scott-Brown M, Alonso-Coello P. Radioisotopes for metastatic bone pain. *Cochrane Database Syst Rev.* 2011;(7):CD003347.
3. Wallace AN, Greenwood TJ, Jennings JW. Radiofrequency ablation and vertebral augmentation for palliation of painful spinal metastases. *J Neurooncol.* 2015;124(1):111-118.
4. Chow E, Zeng L, Salvo N, et al. Update on the systematic review of palliative radiotherapy trials for bone metastases. *Clin Oncol (R Coll Radiol).* 2012;24(2):112-124.
5. Hernandez RK, Adhia A, Wade SW, et al. Prevalence of bone metastases and bone-targeting agent use among solid tumor patients in the United States. *Clin Epidemiol.* 2015;7:335-345.
6. Levy J, Hopkins T, Morris J, et al. Radiofrequency ablation for the palliative treatment of bone metastases: outcomes from the multicenter OsteoCool Tumor Ablation Post-Market Study (OPuS One Study) in 100 patients. *J Vasc Interv Radiol.* 2020;31(11):1745-1752.
7. van der Linden YM, Steenland E, van Houwelingen HC, et al. Patients with a favourable prognosis are equally palliated with single and multiple fraction radiotherapy: results on survival in the Dutch Bone Metastasis Study. *Radiother Oncol.* 2006;78(3):245-253.
8. Berenson J, Pflugmacher R, Jarzem P, et al. Balloon kyphoplasty versus non-surgical fracture management for treatment of painful vertebral body compression fractures in patients with cancer: a multicentre, randomized controlled trial. *Lancet Oncol.* 2011;12(3):225-235.
9. Mannion RJ, Woolf CJ. Pain mechanisms and management: a central perspective. *Clin J Pain.* 2000;16(suppl 3):S144-S156.
10. Goldberg SN, Dupuy DE. Image-guided radiofrequency tumor ablation: challenges and opportunities—part I. *J Vasc Interv Radiol.* 2001;12(9):1021-1032.
11. Goldberg SN. Radiofrequency tumor ablation: principles and techniques. *Eur J Ultrasound.* 2001;13(2):129-147.
12. Rossi S, Stasi MD, Buscarini E, et al. Percutaneous RF interstitial thermal ablation in the treatment of hepatic cancer. *American Journal of Roentgenology.* 1996;196:759-768.
13. National Comprehensive Cancer Network. Clinical Practice Guidelines in Oncology. https://www.nccn.org/professionals/physician_gls/pdf/pain.pdf.
14. Yoon JT, Nesbitt J, Raynor BL, et al. Utility of motor and somatosensory evoked potentials for neural thermoprotection in ablations of musculoskeletal tumors. *J Vasc Interv Radiol.* 2020;31(6):903-911.
15. Buy X, Tok CH, Szwarc D, Bierry G, Gangi A. Thermal protection during percutaneous thermal ablation procedures: interest of carbon dioxide dissection and temperature monitoring. *Cardiovasc Intervent Radiol.* 2009;32(3):529-534.
16. Medtronic. *Osteocool Radiofrequency Ablation System.* https://www.medtronic.com/us-en/healthcare-professionals/products/spinal-orthopaedic/tumor-management/osteocool-ablation-system-rf.html, 2019.
17. Merit Medical. *STARTM Ablation System.* 2022. https://www.merit.com/merit-spine/advanced-energy/ablation/star-tumor-ablation-system/, 2022.
18. Klass D, Marshall T, Toms A. CT-guided radiofrequency ablation of spinal osteoid osteomas with concomitant perineural and epidural irrigation for neuroprotection. *Eur Radiol.* 2009;19(9):2238-2243.
19. Huntoon K, Eltobgy M, Mohyeldin A, Elder JB. Lower extremity paralysis after radiofrequency ablation of vertebral metastases. *World Neurosurg.* 2020;133:178-184.
20. Bagla S, Sayed D, Smirniotopoulos J, et al. Multicenter prospective clinical series evaluating radiofrequency ablation in the treatment of painful spine metastases. *Cardiovasc Intervent Radiol.* 2016;39(9):1289-1297.
21. Greenwood TJ, Wallace A, Friedman MV, et al. Combined ablation and radiation therapy of spinal metastases: a novel multimodality treatment approach. *Pain Physician.* 2015;18(6):573-581.
22. Di Staso M, Zugaro L, Gravina GL, et al. A feasibility study of percutaneous radiofrequency ablation followed by radiotherapy in the management of painful osteolytic bone metastases. *Eur Radiol.* 2011;21(9):2004-2010.

Chapter 9

Basivertebral Nerve Ablation

Alaa Abd-Elsayed and Ahish Chitneni

Introduction

One of the most common health conditions worldwide is chronic low back pain (CLBP). In fact, the point prevalence of low back pain is noted to be around 12% to 33% in the general population.[1] In addition to the pain burden, back pain also is one of the leading causes of disability in the world, affecting over 600 million patients, and is one of the primary leading causes of financial burden on the health care system.[1-3] In order to treat back pain, a stepwise approach is typically taken. Initially, nonpharmacological methods such as education, increased activity, and improvement of posture are all methods that are initiated.[4,5] In addition to education, the use of pharmacological therapies such as analgesic medication are first-line therapy.[5] If conservative measures fail, interventional approaches to the treatment of back pain can be done, such as the use of spinal cord stimulation (SCS) and spinal surgery for patients who may qualify.[5] Many clinical theories exist regarding the source of low back pain. Initially, many theories postulated that over time, as vertebral discs degenerate, the nociceptors in the annulus fibrosus are the primary contributing factor of low back pain.[6] Although for many years this was the prevailing theory, new research has theorized that the basivertebral nerve (BVN) may play a role in carrying nociceptive signals from vertebral end plates that are damaged and result in CLBP.[7] Given the potential for the BVN to result in chronic back pain, effectively localizing and targeting the BVN and conducting a BVN ablation can lead to the resolution of chronic back pain.

Anatomical Considerations

The innervation of the vertebral body by the BVN has been extensively studied by Antonacci et al.

and Fras et al.[8,9] In the study, 69 vertebral bodies were stained for substance P in addition to the nerves innervating the vertebral bodies. The BVN is a branch of the sinuvertebral nerve, which arises from the dorsal root ganglion (DRG). Specifically, the sinuvertebral nerve arises from the ventral ramus of the spinal nerves bilaterally and enters the spinal canal through the basivertebral foramen. In the basivertebral foramen, both BVN and basivertebral plexus travel through the foramen to reach the vertebral end plates.[10] In Fig. 9.1,[11] the BVN can be

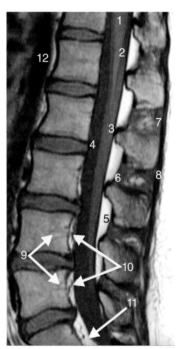

Fig. 9.1 **Basivertebral nerve plexus (#9).** (From Shanechi AM, Kiczek M, Khan M, Jindal G. Spine anatomy imaging: an update. *Neuroimaging Clin N Am.* 2019;29(4):461-480.)

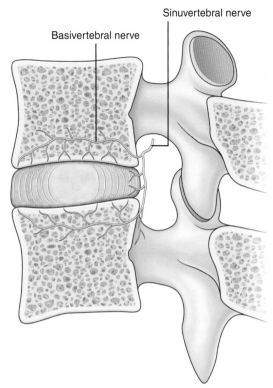

Fig. 9.2 Basivertebral nerve arising from the sinuvertebral nerve.

seen traveling through the basivertebral foramen and innervating the vertebral body. In Fig. 9.2,[7] the sinuvertebral nerve is branching out into the BVN, which innervates the vertebral body.

Patient Selection and Indications

Various patients may qualify to undergo BVN ablation for the treatment of CLBP. First, CLBP as a result of vertebrogenic causes is the number one indication for BVN ablation. As explained earlier, the BVN has been studied as the nerve that innervates the vertebral body. Prior to the conduction of the procedure, other causes of CLBP—such as musculoskeletal conditions, facet joint conditions, and annulus fibrosus trauma must be ruled out. All patients undergoing the procedure must have had CLBP for longer than 6 months that was nonresponsive to at least 3 months of conservative medical care.[12] Additionally, all patients undergoing

the procedure must have no spinal stenosis present and have Type 1 or type 2 Modic changes present on magnetic resonance imaging (MRI).[13] Type 1 and type 2 Modic changes on imaging refers to hypotensive on T1WI and hyperintense on T2WI and hyperintense on T1WI and isointense or slightly hyperintense on T2WI, respectively (Fig. 9.3).[14]

Contraindications

Various contraindications exist that may exclude a patient from undergoing a BVN ablation. In general, patients that have any signs of infection—both systemic and spinal—are typically contraindicated to undergo an interventional spine procedure such as BVN ablation. Other conditions that are contraindications to undergoing this procedure include patients with a spinal malignancy, metastatic malignancy, increased risk of bleeding, pregnancy, and implanted cardiac devices, such as pacemakers.[12,15,16]

Description of Procedure

The BVN ablation procedure is typically performed in an outpatient setting. First, the patient should be positioned prone on the operating table. Patients undergo the procedure under general anesthesia or monitored anesthesia care (MAC) with continuous monitoring.[10] After the patient is placed in a prone position and under anesthesia, the area is prepped in a sterile fashion with the target pedicle and area of entry marked. In general, 1% lidocaine anesthetic is used at the site of entry and an incision is made with the use of a scalpel.[10] Next, an introducer trocar cannula is advanced through the pedicle to enter the posterior vertebral wall, as seen in Fig. 9.4.[17] As the trocar is introduced into the posterior vertebral wall with the use of a mallet, various anteroposterior and C-arm views are obtained to ensure the proper trajectory of the trocar. After ensuring proper trajectory, the introducer trocar is replaced with a curved nitinol stylet probe which allows for the facilitation of a curved path from the posterior vertebral wall to the BVN terminus in the vertebral body, as seen in Fig. 9.5.[17] After fluoroscopic imaging has confirmed the location of the curved stylet, the stylet is replaced with a bipolar radiofrequency probe that is positioned

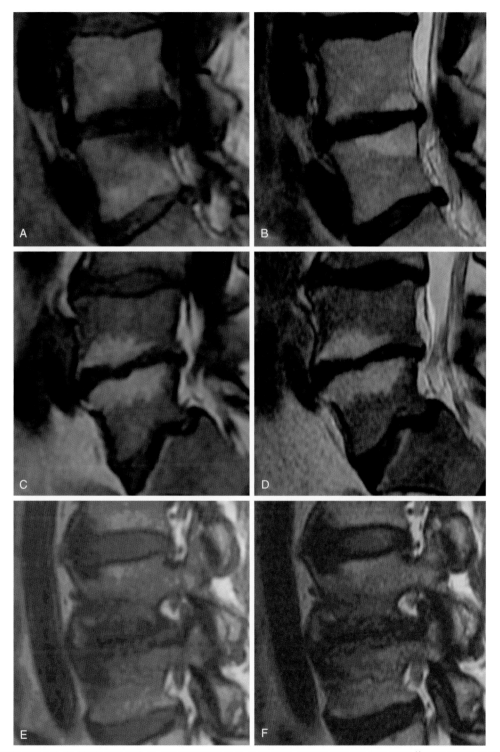

Fig. 9.3 Modic type 1 (A, B), Modic type 2 (C, D), and Modic type 3 (E, F) changes on T1W (*left*) and T2W (*right*).[14] (From Määttä JH, Karppinen JI, Luk KD, Cheung KM, Samartzis D. Phenotype profiling of Modic changes of the lumbar spine and its association with other MRI phenotypes: a large-scale population-based study. *Spine J.* 2015;15(9):1933-1942.)

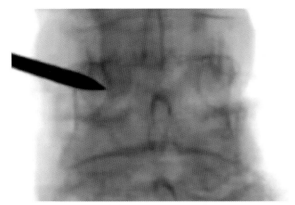

Fig. 9.4 Transversing the pedicle. (From Khalil JG, Smuck M, Koreckij T, et al. A prospective, randomized, multicenter study of intraosseous basivertebral nerve ablation for the treatment of chronic low back pain. *Spine J.* 2019;19(10): 1620–1632.)

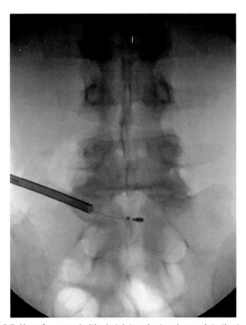

Fig. 9.5 Use of a curved nitinol stylet probe to advance into the terminus of the basivertebral nerve. (From Khalil JG, Smuck M, Koreckij T, et al. A prospective, randomized, multicenter study of intraosseous basivertebral nerve ablation for the treatment of chronic low back pain. *Spine J.* 2019;19(10):1620-1632.)

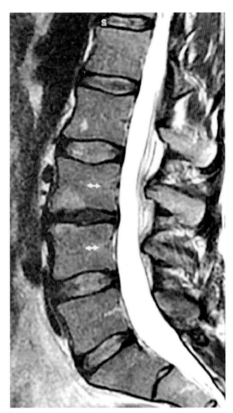

Fig. 9.6 Radiofrequency ablation probe placement location 30% to 50% across the vertebral body width from the posterior wall. (From Khalil JG, Smuck M, Koreckij T, et al. A prospective, randomized, multicenter study of intraosseous basivertebral nerve ablation for the treatment of chronic low back pain. *Spine J.* 2019;19(10):1620-1632.)

similarly at the terminus of the BVN in the vertebral body as seen in Fig. 9.5.[17] The target zone of the probe placement is typically 30% to 50% across the vertebral body width, as seen in Fig. 9.6. After proper placement is confirmed, the radiofrequency probe is activated for 15 minutes at a temperature of 85° C until the creation of a 1-cm lesion in the vertebral body, as seen in Fig. 9.7. After proper ablation, the radiofrequency probe is removed from the vertebral body and the skin is sutured in a sterile fashion.

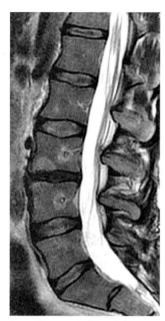

Fig. 9.7 Six weeks posttreatment with radiofrequency ablation. (From Khalil JG, Smuck M, Koreckij T, et al. A prospective, randomized, multicenter study of intraosseous basivertebral nerve ablation for the treatment of chronic low back pain. *Spine J.* 2019;19(10):1620-1632.)

Intraoperative Complications

Given the nature of the procedure, various complications can potentially occur during a BVN ablation. In many of the studies conducted, adverse effects during the procedure were noted to be extremely rare. Despite the rarity of complications, some severe adverse events reported in a systematic review of the procedure included radiculopathy, vertebral compression fracture, retroperitoneal hemorrhage, nerve root injury, spinal hematoma, mild incisional pain, and lower extremity paresthesias.[18,19]

Postoperative Care

Typical postoperative care for radiofrequency ablation procedures includes the application of an adhesive bandage at the puncture site. After the completion of the procedure, the patient is typically transferred to a recovery room for monitoring over the course of the next 15 minutes to 1 hour, with vital signs observed. During this process, the patient is also monitored for

signs of allergic reactions to local medication used. Patients are advised to avoid driving or operating machinery for 24 hours, to avoid any rigorous physical activity for 24 hours, and to remove the adhesive bandage at the puncture site 24 hours postoperatively.[20] Postoperative pain at the puncture site can be managed with the use of an ice pack, nonsteroidal anti-inflammatory drugs, and other over-the-counter medications. Patients are typically discharged on the same day of the procedure, with scheduled postprocedure follow-ups.[10]

General Considerations

Various studies have been conducted on the use of BVN ablation for the treatment of CLBP secondary to vertebrogenic causes. One of the first initial studies conducted was a pilot study by Becker et al.[21] They conducted a single-arm, open-label, human pilot study to determine the efficacy and safety of the BVN ablation procedure. A total of 17 patients with over 6 months of CLBP and Modic type 1 or type 2 changes on MRI were enrolled to receive treatment. Prior to the procedure, baseline measurements of the Oswestry Disability Index (ODI) and Visual Analog Scale (VAS) were recorded at 52 and 61, respectively. After the completion of the ablation, statistically significant improvements in both outcome measures were noted 3 months postprocedure. Results showed that ODI decreased approximately 29 points from the average.[21] Another study was conducted, the SMART trial, by Fischgrund et al.[15] They presented the 2-year clinical outcomes for CLBP patients treated with BVN ablation in a randomized controlled trial. In the study, a total of 147 patients were treated with radiofrequency ablation of the BVN with follow-up through self-assessments; neurological examinations; and safety profile testing at 2 weeks, 6 weeks, 3 months, 6 months, 18 months, and 24 months postoperatively. The ODI and VAS were used as primary outcome measures. Results showed that at 2 years postoperatively, there was a mean percentage improvement of 53.7% and 52.9% in the ODI and VAS scales, respectively, in the BVN group as compared with the sham group.[15] Subjects in the study also had a significant decrease in opioid use and spine injection treatment at the 2-year mark. The INTRACEPT trial, conducted by Khalil et al., also studied the use of BVN ablation.[22] The purpose was to compare the effectiveness of radiofrequency ablation of the BVN compared with standard care for the treatment of CLBP in patients with vertebrogenic-related back pain. In the study, the inclusion criteria for all 140 patients included CLBP for at least 6 months and Modic type 1 or type 2 vertebral end plate changes in the L3 to S1 segments. Patients were randomized to receive radiofrequency ablation of the BVN or standard care. Primary outcome measures for the study included the ODI and VAS, which were collected at baseline and 3, 6, 9, and 12 months postoperatively. In this study, interim analysis showed a clear statistical superiority in the treatment arm compared with the standard care arm. As a result, enrollment for the study was halted at the 3-month mark and crossover to the treatment group was offered to all study participants.[21] In addition, at the 3-month primary end point, results showed that the mean change in ODI in the treatment group was −25.3 compared with −4.4 in the standard care group, whereas the mean change in VAS was −3.46 in the treatment group compared with −1.02 in the standard of care group.

REFERENCES

1. Hoy D, Bain C, Williams G, et al. A systematic review of the global prevalence of low back pain. *Arthritis Rheum.* 2012;64(6):2028-2037.
2. James SL, Abate D, Abate KH, et al. Global, regional, and national incidence, prevalence, and years lived with disability for 354 diseases and injuries for 195 countries and territories, 1990–2017: a systematic analysis for the Global Burden of Disease Study 2017. *Lancet.* 2018;392(10159):1789-1858.
3. Dagenais S, Caro J, Haldeman S. A systematic review of low back pain cost of illness studies in the United States and internationally. *Spine J.* 2008;8(1):8-20.
4. Koes BW, van Tulder MW, Thomas S. Diagnosis and treatment of low back pain. *BMJ.* 2006;332(7555):1430-1434.
5. Al-Kaisy A, Van Buyten JP, Kapural L, et al. 10 kHz spinal cord stimulation for the treatment of non-surgical refractory back pain: subanalysis of pooled data from two prospective studies. *Anaesthesia.* 2020;75(6):775-784.
6. Manchikanti L, Singh V, Pampati V, et al. Evaluation of the relative contributions of various structures in chronic low back pain. *Pain Physician.* 2001;4(4):308-316.
7. Kim HS, Wu PH, Jang IT. Lumbar degenerative disease Part 1: anatomy and pathophysiology of intervertebral discogenic pain

8. Antonacci MD, Mody DR, Heggeness MH. Innervation of the human vertebral body: a histologic study. *J Spinal Disord.* 1998;11(6):526-531.
9. Fras C, Kravetz P, Mody DR, Heggeness MH. Substance P-containing nerves within the human vertebral body. an immunohistochemical study of the basivertebral nerve. *Spine J.* 2003;3(1):63-67.
10. Tieppo FV, Sayed D. *Basivertebral Nerve Ablation.* Treasure Island, FL: StatPearls Publishing; 2021.
11. Shanechi AM, Kiczek M, Khan M, Jindal G. Spine anatomy imaging: an update. *Neuroimaging Clin N Am.* 2019;29(4):461-480.
12. Urits I, Noor N, Johal AS, et al. Basivertebral nerve ablation for the treatment of vertebrogenic pain. *Pain Ther.* 2021;10(1):39-53.
13. Modic MT, Steinberg PM, Ross JS, Masaryk TJ, Carter JR. Degenerative disk disease: assessment of changes in vertebral body marrow with MR imaging. *Radiology.* 1988;166(1 Pt 1):193-199.
14. Määttä JH, Karppinen JI, Luk KD, Cheung KM, Samartzis D. Phenotype profiling of Modic changes of the lumbar spine and its association with other MRI phenotypes: a large-scale population-based study. *Spine J.* 2015;15(9):1933-1942.
15. Fischgrund JS, Rhyne A, Franke J, et al. Intraosseous basivertebral nerve ablation for the treatment of chronic low back pain: 2-year results from a prospective randomized double-blind sham-controlled multicenter study. *Int J Spine Surg.* 2019;13(2):110-119.
16. Lorio M, Clerk-Lamalice O, Beall DP, Julien T. International Society for the Advancement of Spine Surgery guideline—intraosseous ablation of the basivertebral nerve for the relief of chronic low back pain. *Int J Spine Surg.* 2020;14(1):18-25.
17. Fischgrund JS, Rhyne A, Franke J, et al. Intraosseous basivertebral nerve ablation for the treatment of chronic low back pain: a prospective randomized double-blind sham-controlled multicenter study. *Eur Spine J.* 2018;27:1146-1156.
18. Tieppo FV, Sherwood D, Twohey E, et al. Developments in minimally invasive surgical options for vertebral pain: basivertebral nerve ablation—a narrative review. *J Pain Res.* 2021;14:1887-1907.
19. Conger A, Schuster NM, Cheng DS, et al. The effectiveness of intraosseous basivertebral nerve radiofrequency neurotomy for the treatment of chronic low back pain in patients with modic changes: a systematic review. *Pain Med.* 2021;22(5):1039-1054.
20. Radiofrequency ablation. Cleveland Clinic. Radiofrequency ablation. https://my.clevelandclinic.org/health/treatments/17411-radiofrequency-ablation. Accessed December 16, 2021.
21. Becker S, Hadjipavlou A, Heggeness MH. Ablation of the basivertebral nerve for treatment of back pain: a clinical study. *Spine J.* 2017;17:218-223.
22. Khalil JG, Smuck M, Koreckij T, et al. A prospective, randomized, multicenter study of intraosseous basivertebral nerve ablation for the treatment of chronic low back pain. *Spine J.* 2019;19(10):1620-1632.

Chapter 10

Outcome Measurement for Vertebral Augmentation

Manuchehr Habibi, Joshua M. Martens, and Alaa Abd-Elsayed

Introduction

The prevalence of spine fractures in the United States was estimated to be 11% in people 70 to 79 years old and 18% in those over 80 years of age.[1] With the increasing morbidity and diminished quality of life resulting from these fractures, percutaneous vertebral body augmentation procedures have become a favorable treatment option by many providers and interventionists.[2] Vertebral augmentation is a minimally invasive procedure that involves the injection of polymethylmethacrylate (PMMA) into the vertebral body to internally stabilize it, leading to pain relief.[3] As with any procedure, in order to improve the intervention or continue to recommend it, a measurement of outcomes should be a cornerstone.

Measuring outcomes aids in improving the efficacy and efficiency of a procedure. It allows utilization of the data as evidence for clinical decisions and selecting the best-fitted intervention for a patient.[4] Furthermore, it promotes the adoption of best practices[5] and creates an opportunity for further research. It is vital to recognize that defining pre- and post–Visual Analog Scale (VAS) pain scores may not be sufficient for outcome measurement and that other metrics, such as disability and quality of life changes, also need to be included. After all, the primary aim should be to improve the patient's quality of life and well-being.[5] Before considering vertebral augmentation, the careful selection of a patient, as discussed in Chapter 2, is a critical step for the success and better outcomes of the procedure.

Outcome Measurement Components and Tools

A careful history, pain score, and characterization of pain are prudent to obtain during the first patient encounter. In addition, a history of prior treatments, surgeries, their efficacy, personal medical history, and medications are a valuable addition to the decision-making process. There are multiple tools available to clinicians that can aid in assessing the patient's pain, quality of life, physical limitations, and psychological impact of the disease. Some of the most commonly used instruments are summarized next, grouped by pain, disability, and quality of life.

1. Visual Analog Scale (VAS)[6]
   A. Publicly available scale.
   B. Measures pain intensity and is suitable for a broad range of ages.
   C. Scores are self-reported with a mark on a 10-cm line representing a continuum of "no pain" at the zero mark and "the worst pain" at the 10-cm mark.
   D. The scale can be downloaded from many sources online or made manually.
2. Brief Pain Inventory (BPI)
   A. It is a proprietary questionnaire that assesses the severity of both malignant and nonmalignant pain and their impact on daily functions.[7]

B. This instrument measures seven domains: general activity, mood, walking ability, normal work, relations with others, sleep, and enjoyment of life. The scale ranges from 0 to 10.[7]

C. The form can be ordered from https://www.mdanderson.org/symptomresearch/index.cfm.

3. McGill Pain Questionnaire

A. A questionnaire that was developed by Dr. Melzack at McGill University in Montreal, Canada that helps describe the pain a patient is experiencing and translate it to a numerical score.[8]

B. The minimum score is 0 and the maximum score is 78. The higher the score, the more severe the pain.[8]

C. A publicly available version can be downloaded from the following link: https://www.sralab.org/sites/default/files/2017-07/McGill%20Pain%20Questionnaire%20%281%29.pdf.

4. Roland-Morris Disability Questionnaire (RMDQ)

A. Publicly available

B. It measures disability consisting of a total of 24 items that can be marked or not. Every item that is not marked is counted as zero. The higher scores represent a higher level of disability.[9]

C. A change of 2 to 3 points from the baseline is considered significant.[9-11]

D. The form can be downloaded for free from http://www.rmdq.org/Download.htm.

5. Oswestry Disability Index (ODI)

A. It is used to assess pain-related disability with low back pain (most commonly in patients with severe symptoms).[12]

B. Two versions of the ODI questionnaire are available. The original version 1.0 has been adopted by the American Academy of Orthopaedic Surgeons (AAOS) whereas Version 2.0 has been more widely used in the United Kingdom.[12]

C. Each question has a possible 5 points with a total score of 50, which is interpreted as completely disabled.

D. Version 1.0 can be downloaded from https://aaos.org/globalassets/quality-and-

practice-resources/patient-reported-outcome-measures/spine/oswestry-2.pdf.

6. Short Form 36 Health Survey Questionnaire (SF-36)

A. The most widely used tool that measures the health status and the quality of life.

B. The scale provides a measure of the physical and mental components of health. It reflects eight domains of health: physical function, bodily pain, role limitations due to physical health problems, role limitations due to personal or emotional problems, general mental health, social functioning, energy/fatigue or vitality, and general health perceptions.[13]

C. A licensed revised version can be found from Optum Incorporated (https://cdn-aem.optum.com/content/dam/optum/resources/Manual%20Excerpts/SF-36v2_Manual_Chapter_1.pdf) and a publicly available version of the SF-36 with scoring instructions can be downloaded from the following link: https://www.rand.org/health-care/surveys_tools/mos/36-item-short-form/scoring.html.

7. Karnofsky Performance Status (KPS) Scale

A. This is a frequently used scale for quantifying the functional status of cancer patients.[14]

B. The scale goes from 0 (dead) to 100 (normal without evidence of disease).[14]

C. A publicly available version can be downloaded from http://www.npcrc.org/files/news/karnofsky_performance_scale.pdf.

8. EuroQoL-5 (EQ5D)[15]

A. It is a fee-based tool to assess a patient's quality of life.

B. The 5L version assesses five dimensions: mobility, self-care, usual activities, pain/discomfort, and anxiety/depression. Each dimension has three levels: no problems, moderate problems, severe problems.[16] A summary index with a maximum score of 1 indicates the best health state.[17]

C. The fee-based version can be downloaded from https://euroqol.org/support/how-to-obtain-eq-5d/.

9. Quality of Life for Osteoporosis (QUALEFFO-41)[18]

A. Publicly available questionnaire to assess the quality of life in patients with osteoporosis.

B. The survey consists of seven domains: pain, activities of daily living, jobs around the house, mobility, leisure and social activities, general health perception, and mental function.

C. A scoring algorithm can be found from https://www.osteoporosis.foundation/sites/iofbonehealth/files/2020-01/Qualeffo-Scoring-Algorithm.pdf.

D. The free version can be downloaded from https://www.osteoporosis.foundation/health-professionals/research-tools/quality-life-questionnaires.

10. Tokuhashi Score

A. Used for preoperative evaluation of a patient's prognosis with a metastatic spinal tumor. A revised score from 2017 has been shown to have an improved prognostic ability.[19,20]

B. The tool consists of five domains: general condition (based on Karnofsky Performance Status Scale), number of metastases in the vertebral body, metastases to the major internal organs, the primary site of the cancer, and state of paralysis. A score of 0 to 5 represents < 6 months' mean survival period, 6 to 8 more than 6 months, and 9 to 12 more than 12 months.[20]

C. Some studies recommend vertebroplasty for a score of 4 or less.[21]

D. A publicly available version can be found from the following link: https://link.springer.com/article/10.1007/s00432-017-2519-y/tables/4.

In order for the outcomes to be relevant, a vertebral augmentation intervention must be deemed successful. A technical and procedural success can be defined as appropriate vertebral height change[22]; absence of inadequately filled fractures[23]; cement reaching the posterior fourth of the vertebral body[10]; absence of an epidural, foraminal, or venous leakage[24]; an absence of any immediate postprocedural complications, such as infection, cord compression, or hemodynamic instability, including cardiac perforation,[25] allergic reactions, and pulmonary embolism.[24]

Patients who have undergone successful invasive treatment interventions are followed up closely to monitor their response to therapy. The timing of follow-up is not clearly defined, but several studies implemented 1 to 2 weeks for short-term[26] and 12 to 24 months for long-term follow up.[23] The follow-up includes assessing the ability to resume and maintain activities of daily living such as self-care, housework, family and leisure activities, improvement in anxiety and depression scores, and adverse events.[27,28] In addition, measurement of postprocedure VAS score and, equally important, physical and quality of life improvement, may be necessary to determine whether the intervention was efficacious when compared with preintervention baseline scores. It would also be helpful to collect information through imaging on the subsequent or adjacent vertebral fracture or re-fractures at the treated level.[23,28,29] In summary, during the initial patient encounter, obtaining a thorough history that includes prior interventions and their efficacy, updated imaging for characterization of the vertebral deformities, and answers to the pain, quality-of-life and disability questionnaires is key to starting a patient on a path to freedom from the debilitating effects of osteoporotic vertebral fractures. Moreover, it is important to recognize that there is no single instrument that can be utilized to evaluate results following an osteoporotic vertebral fracture intervention. A combination of surveys building an overall health assessment picture is the recommended approach.[30]

REFERENCES

1. Cosman F, Krege JH, Looker AC, et al. Spine fracture prevalence in a nationally representative sample of US women and men aged ≥ 40 years: results from the National Health and Nutrition Examination Survey (NHANES) 2013–2014. *Osteoporos Int.* 2017;28(6):1857-1866.

2. Goz V, Errico TJ, Weinreb JH, et al. Vertebroplasty and kyphoplasty: national outcomes and trends in utilization from 2005 through 2010. *Spine J.* 2015;15(5):959-965.

3. Garfin SR, Reilley MA. Minimally invasive treatment of osteoporotic vertebral body compression fractures. *Spine J.* 2002;2(1):76-80.

4. Ching S, Thoma A, McCabe RE, Antony MM. Measuring outcomes in aesthetic surgery: a comprehensive review of the literature. *Plast Reconstr Surg.* 2003;111(1):469-482.

5. Pantaleon L. Why measuring outcomes is important in health care. *J Vet Intern Med.* 2019;33(2):356-362.

6. Delgado DA, Lambert BS, Boutris N, et al. Validation of digital visual analog scale pain scoring with a traditional paper-based visual analog scale in adults. *J Am Acad Orthop.* 2018;2(3):e088.

7. Tan G, Jensen MP, Thornby JI, Shanti BF. Validation of the Brief Pain Inventory for chronic nonmalignant pain. *J Pain.* 2004;5(2):133-137.

8. Melzack R. The McGill Pain Questionnaire: major properties and scoring methods. *Pain.* 2018;1(3):277-299.

9. Stratford PW, Riddle DL. A Roland Morris Disability Questionnaire target value to distinguish between functional and dysfunctional states in people with low back pain. *Physiother Can.* 2016;68(1):29-35.

10. Trout AT, Kallmes DF, Gray LA, Goodnature BA, et al. Evaluation of vertebroplasty with a validated outcome measure: the Roland-Morris Disability Questionnaire. *AJNR Am J Neuroradiol.* 2005;26(10):2652-2657.

11. Roland M, Fairbank J. The Roland–Morris disability questionnaire and the Oswestry disability questionnaire. *Spine.* 2000;25(24):3115-3124.

12. Fairbank JC, Pynsent PB. The Oswestry Disability Index. *Spine.* 2000;25(22):2940-2953.

13. Ware JE Jr. SF-36 health survey update. *Spine.* 2000;25(24):3130-3139.

14. Schag CC, Heinrich RL, Ganz PA. Karnofsky performance status revisited: reliability, validity, and guidelines. *J Clin Oncol.* 1984;2(3):187-193.

15. Group TE. EuroQol—a new facility for the measurement of health-related quality of life. *Health Policy.* 1990;16(3):199-208.

16. Obradovic M, Lal A, Liedgens H. Validity and responsiveness of EuroQol-5dimension (EQ-5D) versus Short Form-6 dimension (SF-6D) questionnaire in chronic pain. *Health Qual Life Outcomes.* 2016;11(1):1-9.

17. EuroQol Research Foundation. *EQ-5D-5L User Guide.* 2019. https://euroqol.org/publications/user-guides. Accessed September 10, 2022.

18. Lips P, Cooper C. *Qualeffo-41 Scoring Algorithm (January 2020).* n.d. https://www.osteoporosis.foundation/health-professionals/research-tools/quality-life-questionnaires. Accessed September 10, 2022.

19. Tokuhashi Y, Uei H, Oshima M, Ajiro Y. Scoring system for prediction of metastatic spine tumor prognosis. *World J Orthop.* 2014;5(3):262.

20. Morgen SS, Fruergaard S, Gehrchen M, Bjørck S, Engelholm, SA, Dahl B. A revision of the Tokuhashi revised score improves the prognostic ability in patients with metastatic spinal cord compression. *J Cancer Res Clin Oncol.* 2018;144(1):33-38.

21. Alvarez L, Perez-Higueras A, Quinones D, Calvo E, Rossi RE. Vertebroplasty in the treatment of vertebral tumors: postprocedural outcome and quality of life. *Eur Spine J.* 2003;12(4):356-360.

22. Trumm CG, Jakobs TF, Stahl R, et al. CT fluoroscopy-guided vertebral augmentation with a radiofrequency-induced, high-viscosity bone cement (StabiliT®): technical results and polymethylmethacrylate leakages in 25 patients. *Skelet Radiol.* 2013;42(1):113-120.

23. Jacobson RE, Palea O, Granville M. Progression of vertebral compression fractures after previous vertebral augmentation: technical reasons for recurrent fractures in a previously treated vertebra. *Cureus.* 2017;9(10):e1776.

24. Cohen JE, Lylyk P, Ceratto R, Kaplan L, Umansky F, Gomori JM. Percutaneous vertebroplasty: technique and results in 192 procedures. *Neurol Res.* 2004;26(1):41-49.

25. Al-Nakshabandi NA. Percutaneous vertebroplasty complications. *Ann Saudi Med.* 2011;31(3):294-297.

26. Hatgis J, Granville M, Jacobson RE. Evaluation and interventional management of pain after vertebral augmentation procedures. *Cureus.* 2017;9(2):e1061.

27. Garfin SR, Reilley MA. Minimally invasive treatment of osteoporotic vertebral body compression fractures. *Spine J.* 2002;2(1):76-80.

28. Farrokhi MR, Alibai E, Maghami Z. Randomized controlled trial of percutaneous vertebroplasty versus optimal medical management for the relief of pain and disability in acute osteoporotic vertebral compression fractures. *J Neurosurg Spine.* 2011;14(5):561-569.

29. Boonen S, Van Meirhaeghe J, Bastian L, et al. Balloon kyphoplasty for the treatment of acute vertebral compression fractures: 2-year results from a randomized trial. *J Bone Miner Res.* 2011;26(7):1627-1637.

30. Schoenfeld AJ, Bono CM. Measuring spine fracture outcomes: common scales and checklists. *Injury.* 2011;42(3):265-270.

INDEX

Page numbers followed by "f" and "t" indicate figures and tables respectively.